The

10 Compelling Reasons to Choose a Plant-based Diet & Lifestyle

The Why & The How

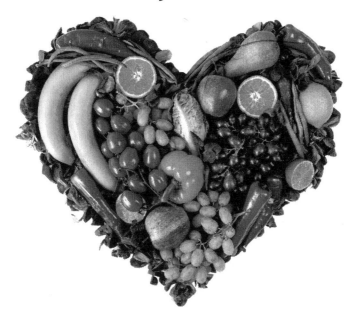

★ Be Vibrantly Healthy
★ Prevent Future Pandemics
★ Reverse the Climate Crisis
★ Eliminate Starvation
★ Lovingkindness to All Animals
★ Elevate Your Consciousness
★ Enjoy Signature Recipes

Meenakshi Angel Honig

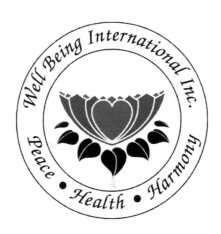

© 2022 Meenakshi Honig

All rights reserved. No part of this book may be used or reproduced in any manner whatsoever without the expressed written permission of the author.

Address all inquiries to Wellbeing International, Inc.

Email: Angel@AngelYoga.com

Website: www.AngelYoga.com

Wellbeing International, Inc.
PO Box 2300
Kihei, Hawaii 96753

ISBN: 978-1-889348-02-5

Library of Congress Control Number: 2021924504

Endorsements from Global Experts & New York Times Bestselling Authors for *The Soulution* by Meenakshi Angel Honig

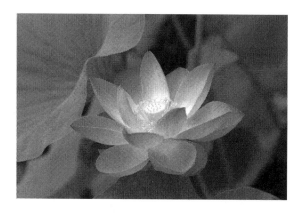

"This book is a game-changer! *The Soulution* brilliantly shows how our dietary choices impact every aspect of life and offers a path to healing ourselves, the animals and our planet. Meenakshi Angel Honig's step-by-step approach moves us from information to implementation to transformation. A beautiful book for these times!"
- **Marci Shimoff, #1 New York Times bestselling author of *Happy For No Reason* & *Love For No Reason***

"What's good for you is good for the planet. What's personally sustainable is globally sustainable. In *The Soulution*, Meenakshi Angel Honig presents why and how."
- **Dean Ornish, M.D., New York Times bestselling author of *Dr. Dean Ornish's Program for Reversing Heart Disease, Eat More, Weigh Less, Love & Survival* & *The Spectrum*, Founder & President of Preventive Medicine Research Institute, Clinical Professor of Medicine, University of California, San Francisco**

"*The Soulution*, by Meenakshi Angel Honig, is an exquisite keyring filled with the shining keys that will unlock a healthier, happier future for us all. No matter which door in your mind or heart you need to be opened to a vegan way of eating and living, *The Soulution* will turn the lock. Are you concerned about your own health? Do you care about the suffering of animals? Do you want to protect the Earth from ruination? How about a livable future for our children?
In this remarkable, readable and resource-filled book, Meenakshi takes on the thorniest of issues and tackles the most obstinate of objections commonly used to justify meat-eating - and she melts them away with logic and love to guide us to a future of sustainability and compassion. Matching every "why to do it" with a "how to do it,"
The Soulution is as practical as it is inspiring - a perfect guide for our time. Accept the gift that is this book, take its message into your heart and watch your life become part of
The Soulution."
- **Michael Klaper, M.D., Author of** *Vegan Nutrition: Pure & Simple* **& Director of Moving Medicine Forward Initiative**

"*The Soulution* is an important new book with a timely message. As climate destruction looms over our futures, everyone in the modern world today must be aware that what they eat does not just control their own health destiny, but the health and future of our planet. Those who are working tirelessly to benefit our planet are the heroes of today. You must be part of *The Soulution*."
- **Joel Fuhrman, M.D., 7-time #1 New York Times bestselling author of** *Eat for Life* **& President of Nutritional Research Foundation**

"In *The Solution*, Meenakshi Angel Honig offers a clear and compelling case for choosing a plant-based diet for your wellbeing, for lovingkindness to all animals, and for the very survival of life on Earth. Angel also includes her signature recipes to make the transition as easy as a 'peace' of vegan cake."
- John Robbins, Bestselling author of *Diet for a New America* & President of The Food Revolution Network

"I would highly recommend this book to everyone. It can help those new to a plant-centered diet, as well as those who are already aware of its benefits. Written with unique clarity and accessibility, it is a book that can not only help in health and healing, but as an inspiration to the remarkable importance of the emerging science of lifestyle medicine."
- Sandra Amrita McLanahan, M.D., Co-author of *Surgery & Its Alternatives*, *Dr. Yoga*, *After Cancer Care* & *Take a Deep Breath*

"Angel's book provides you with the compelling why and how to choose a plant-based diet and lifestyle. It includes; mind set, Angel's signature recipes, resources, a well laid out practical plan for how to make a graceful transition, naturally arrive at your ideal weight, age gracefully, choose cruelty free makeup and household products and so much more! If you want to experience vibrant health, radiant beauty and inner peace at any age, this book is your *Soulution!*"
- Mark Taylor, M.D.

"We are all acutely aware that we're living in a time of unparalleled challenges, and so it is eminently inspiring to read and absorb this new book by Angel Honig that sheds much-needed light on the roots of the problems we are facing. She illuminates ten hidden and far-reaching consequences of the living core of our culture, which is animal agriculture, and clearly elucidates the remarkable practical benefits of questioning the prevailing food narrative. A special bonus in this book is her elegant and enticingly simple and straightforward way of preparing meals that are nutritious, delicious, and that radiate healing energy not just into our bodies, but into our world as well, on every level. You'll want to buy two; one to read and keep close, and one to give to a valued friend."

- Will Tuttle, Ph.D., Bestselling author of *The World Peace Diet*, former Zen monk, inspirational speaker & musician

"If you want healing, vitality and light-filled Qi, (aka chi and prana) flowing through your body and heartmind and you want to have a powerful healing impact on the environment, animals and all of humanity, following the guidance in Meenakshi Angel Honig's new book is your *Soulution*!"

- Dr. Roger Jahnke, OMD., Bestselling author of *The Healer Within, The Healing Promise of Qi*, Founder of Institute of Integral Qigong & Tai Chi & The Healer Within Foundation

"This book is a MUST READ for anyone wanting to raise their vibration, adopt an even juicier plant-based lifestyle, and soar to great heights of health & vitality!"

- Sage Lavine, #1 Bestselling Hay House author of *Women Rocking Business*

"*The Soulution*, by Meenakshi Angel Honig, is a book of encouragement. This beautifully written book could not have come at better time in our lives. It provides a wealth of information for anyone interested in attaining optimal health, protecting animals and saving the environment. If you need a push to become vegan, this ought to do it!"
- **Laurelee Blanchard, Author of *Finding Paradise* & President of Leilani Farm Sanctuary**

"*The Soulution* is a thorough, intelligent, compelling, heartfelt, and stirring illumination and celebration of how to upgrade the quality of our lives and the life of the planet by returning to a natural, plant-based diet. Through many powerful examples and personal testimonials, Meenakshi Angel Honig shows us not just why lightening our diet will help us, but how to achieve it. Anyone reading this gem of a book will be inspired to take the best possible care of yourself while compassionately sharing our world with other living beings. Thank you, Meenakshi, for your courageous and uplifting contribution!"
- **Alan Cohen, Award-winning author of *A Deep Breath of Life***

"Whether you're ready to choose a completely plant-based diet or not, this book lays out a clear step-by-step plan to making healthier food choices. Meenakshi Angel Honig is a master of wholesome nutrition and offers solid, sound advice that is both good for you, for those you love, and for our planet too."
- **Katherine Woodward Thomas, New York Times bestselling author of *Calling in "The One"* & *Conscious Uncoupling***

"*The Soulution* is a comprehensive, inspiring and illuminating wakeup call! Meenakshi Angel Honig provides us with the intelligent and irrefutable why and the easy how to choose a healthy vegan diet and lifestyle. Through her book, your critical thinking left brain, your practical self, your body, your heart and your intuitive Soul's knowing will be activated and engaged. Angel inspires us to make conscious and loving choices that support our health, the animals and our environment. Deepest gratitude to Angel for distilling this vast topic and connecting the dots to provide us with the knowledge, extraordinary resources and step by step plan to make the transition to a vegan lifestyle easy, delicious and doable! I bow to Angel for taking a powerful stand for animal advocacy and for her lifelong dedication to benevolence and to the liberation of all beings."

- **Rebecca McLean, Founder of The Circle of Life Coach Institute, Cofounder of The Healer Within Foundation & Health Action, Inc., Master Board-Certified Life Coach, Certified Qigong & Mindfulness Teacher**

"This book brings answers to the soul—how to heal the soul of the planet, respect the souls of the animals and bring peace and joy to your own soul. Meenakshi Angel Honig identifies and provides *the Soulution* to what is plaguing our world today. In an era of pandemics, the cure is spelled out clearly and succinctly in *The Soulution*."

- **Julie Stuehser, International Diplomat of Light**

"Lovingkindness is at the core of Angel's impassioned plea for a vegan diet. Her message is timely at this moment when our planet is riddled with pandemic and peril. Her message is one of hope for humans, for animals, and for our beloved Mother Earth. Often people try to wiggle out of making hard dietary choices, coming up with a myriad of excuses as to why it just won't work. Angel highlights these common alibis and counters them with reasoned and compassionate replies. In this way, she highlights misconceptions that may stand in the way of a person struggling with how to move forward on the path to becoming a vegan. Angel includes recipes and tips on how to make the transition to a vegan diet both manageable and joyful!"
- **Jiya Kowarsky, Author of *River of Joy***

"Meenakshi Angel Honig has poured her heart, soul and life-long devotion to a Yogic lifestyle–embracing veganism and being a voice for the animals and the environment– into this most compelling and provocative contribution to humanity. This book is a must-read for anyone interested in upgrading the quality of their health and vitality, and contributing to a kinder, gentler, more sustainable world. Thank you, Angel, for the tireless dedication, care and compassion that you spread to the world through your important & masterfully sculpted message. There couldn't be a more important time to share this wisdom with the world than now!"
- **Ashanna Solaris, Co-founder & Pioneer of Clarity Breathwork**

"At our dinner table, as our mother took off the steaming lid covering the roasted Thanksgiving turkey, Angel at age 9 yelled out "Eeeewww that is a dead bird, I am not going to eat that!" On that day, because of her love for animals, Angel became a vegetarian. This was a very courageous move considering that we didn't know even one other vegetarian at that time. Over the years, Angel has helped thousands of people, including our entire family, transition to plant-based nutrition. Angel is a leading proponent of human, animal and environmental wellbeing. She hosts seminars, retreats, classes and personal counseling sessions helping humanity embrace plant-based nutrition and healthy lifestyle choices. She has written a plethora of articles, pamphlets and books on vegan nutrition, including her opus magnum, a nearly 600 page book entitled, *Feel Good Now ~ How to Feel Your Best & Have Your Best to Give*. Angel's newest masterpiece, **The Soulution**, combines her years of research and expertise as a certified Yoga Instructor and Wellbeing Consultant into one book. This landmark book lays out the facts that are undeniable. Anyone reading this book will be touched by its clarity and inspired to embrace a vegan lifestyle that is compassionate to all beings."

- Fredrick Swaroop Honig, Author of *The Scientific Proof of God: Unified Field Theory Revealed*

"These times of great change across the globe invite us all to re-assess our lifestyle choices, both for our personal wellbeing and also for the wellbeing of our planet.
The Soulution is a powerful and yet accessible guide to transforming your health, the wellbeing of animals and our planet, by embracing a plant-based diet. Written from the heart by a vibrant vegan and illuminated Yogini, this book is sure to educate and inspire you, and ultimately support you to embody your own deepest values in this world."
- **Miranda Macpherson, International Spiritual Teacher & bestselling author of *The Way of Grace: The Transforming Power of Ego Relaxation***

"Meenakshi Angel Honig is a loud, clear and compassionate voice for the animals, for human health and for the very survival of our precious planet Earth. Because she fully embodies what she is sharing in ***The Soulution***, the words on these pages are not mere words but rather this book is a transmission that will catalyze a transformation in your thinking, your dietary choices, your health, the evolution of your Soul and the ripple effect of benevolence to all beings and forms of life!"
- **Sarah Taylor, Bestselling author of *Vegan in 30 Days & Vegetarian to Vegan***

"If you are concerned about preventing future pandemics, reversing the climate crisis, eliminating starvation, ending animal cruelty and improving your health, this exemplary book is your ***Soulution***! Meenakshi Angel Honig has created a golden bridge to living the golden rule and ushering in a Golden Age!"
- **Mirabai Devi, Author of *Samadhi: Essence of the Divine*, International Spiritual Teacher & Founder of the Mirabai Devi Foundation**

"Meenakshi's new book is truly an outpouring of her heart's love and an expression of her life's mission. Even as a young girl, she took what was a bold step back then, and gave up eating meat. Her dedication to the protection of all life and to the practice of *ahimsa*, non-violence, comes from her very soul. I have no doubt that her earnest and pure voice to free all beings from suffering will reach the heavens and draw divine blessings on us all."

- *S*wami Karunananda, Bestselling author of *Awakening: Aspiration to Realization Through Integral Yoga* & highly acclaimed Senior Teacher of Integral Yoga International

Acknowledgments

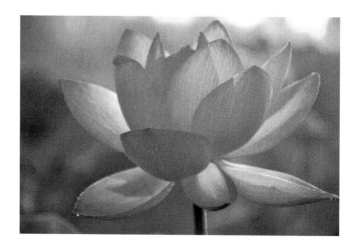

My heartfelt gratitude to these precious beings. Thank you for all of your loving & generous support in countless ways! I would not be who I am & this book would not be what it is, without You!

The Divine Benevolence that abides, guides & glides through me
Master Sivananda
Swami Satchidananda
Jean & Jacob Honig
Jiya Honig Kowarsky
Robert Ram Honig
Edward Lawrence Honig
Fredrick Swaroop Honig
Steve Kowarsky
Rebecca McLean
Vajra Matusow
Swami Karunananda
Madhuri Honeyman
Aerie Waters

Vegan Inspiration ~ Deep gratitude to these noble vegan teachers!

John Robbins
Dr. Michael Klaper
Dr. Will Tuttle
Dr. Dean Ornish
Dr. Sandra Amrita McLanahan
Dr. Michael Greger
Dr. Joel Fuhrman
Dr. Neal Barnard
Bruce Friedrich

Profound gratitude to my vegan kindred spirit, mentor & editor of this book, who is a vibrant embodiment of the vegan message & the author of The *World Peace Diet*, Dr. Will Tuttle.

Loving gratitude to Yana Viniko for your kind & generous *Hands in Hands Partnership* grant to provide complimentary copies of this book for people in undeserved communities.

Thank you to these loving Souls for your support & generous contributions for this book ~ Julie & Reagan Stuehser, Sarah & Mark Taylor, Brook Le'amohala, Kevin Olsen, Lydia Deems, Alan Thompson, Ricardo Dgama & Mina Takayanagi.

Special thanks to Rebecca French for volunteering to help me, side-by-side, to test recipes, navigate through Grammarly, gather & organize photos, proofread, etc. She is a true shining light of Karma Yoga which is the path of selfless service!

I would like to thank James Mylenek Sr. for working with me, side-by-side, to bring my vision for the layout & formatting of each page into actualization with his awe-inspiring technowizardry, diligence, patience, generosity & kind nature!

My sincere gratitude to my teachers, ancestors, family, friends, everyone & everything that has contributed to my wellbeing, to the evolution of my Soul & to the vegan movement.

Thank you to all of my kindred vegan advocates who are helping to make planet Earth a kinder & safer place to be.

Thank **You** for reading, implementing & sharing this message!

I bow in gratitude to the Divine Beloved in all these myriad names & forms.

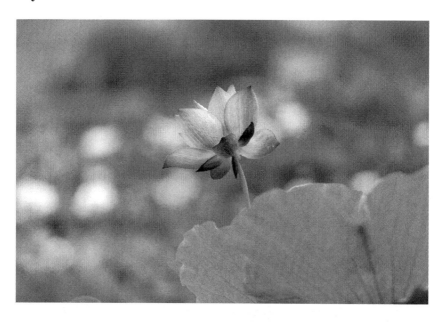

Table of Contents

Endorsements i

Acknowledgements xi

Table of Contents xv

Introduction ~ Light One Small Candle xix

Being a Voice 1

Definitions.. 7

Supercharge Your Wellbeing on All Levels
with the Lovingkindness Diet & Lifestyle 11

Ten Compelling Reasons to Choose a Plant-based Diet.. 15
1) Animal Welfare... 16
2) Eliminate World Hunger & Starvation...................... 20
3) Reverse Water Shortage.. 22
4) Reverse Deforestation 24
5) Reverse Global Warming & The Climate Crisis........ 26
6) Reverse Pollution 32
7) Increase Energy ~ Individual & Global 34
8) Improve Health & Prevent Future Pandemics 36
9) Eliminate Modern Day Slavery & Put an End to War.... 46
10) It Is the Right Thing to Do! 49

The Vital Importance of Transitioning
from Vegetarian to Vegan 53

The Boomerang Effect 65

How to Prevent Future Pandemics.................................... 69

From Dissonance to Consonance ~
From Disconnection to Reconnection 77

Counter Questions Instead of Counter Attacks 83

My Wish to Protect Fish 121

How to Transition to a Plant-Based Diet
with Ease, Grace & Joy 133

Seven Guidelines for Optimum Nutrition 139

Cleansing Diet 147

Feel Great at Your Ideal Weight 153

Graceful Eldering 161

Say No to GMO 169

To Bee or Not to Bee 173

Break Up with Non-Vegan Makeup! 179

Evolution of a Soul 185

Set Yourself Up to Succeed ~
This is not a diet; this is a lifestyle 191

Angel's Basic Template for a Healthy Balanced Diet 201

Honoring the Season & the Life-force 227

Angel's Favorite Go-to Meals 231

Angel's Recipes 237

Declaration of Independence for Animals 319

Conclusion ~ The Power of Love 325

Resources 335

About Angel ~ Services & Products 344

Dedication 355

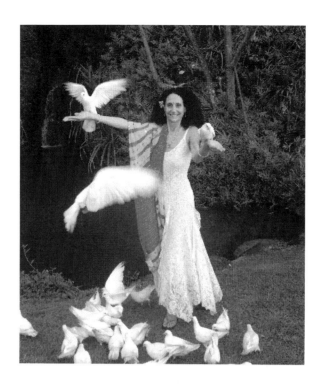

Welcome to *The Soulution*

10 Compelling Reasons to Choose a Plant-based Diet

The Why & The How

"It is better to light a candle than to curse the darkness."
- Confucius

Most people enter into a plant-based lifestyle through one of four main doors: concern for the animals, for the environment, for their health, or for enhanced athletic performance. Whatever door beckons you, welcome! I am glad that you are here!

I am an ethical vegan & entered into this lifestyle because of my love for animals. Then I came to learn of the astounding benefits for the environment, for human health & for wellbeing on all levels!

It is profoundly disturbing to me that for the vast majority of people on planet Earth today, the imprisonment, torture & murder of animals is not a significant issue. People check out in grocery store lines with the flesh & secretions of abused cows, pigs, lambs, chickens, goats & fishes. All of these living beings have real feelings, similar to ours & yet nobody blinks an eye.

People have barbecues & eat hotdogs, hamburgers, pork chops, eggs & dairy products with no regard for the horrific suffering that was inflicted on these animals who can feel pain, as we do.

How can this be? How can it be that good people—loving, caring & seemingly well-educated people, including pet lovers, religious leaders, spiritual teachers & Yoga instructors—can be agents of such gruesome violence & cruelty, as if it were nothing?

It is because most of us have been duped & wounded in what Dr. Will Tuttle, author of *The World Peace Diet*, describes as a "cultural trance."

It is understandable that we have fallen prey to this cultural trance because we have been fed this "food" since we were infants & have followed without questioning what we are doing. We have been conditioned to think that this is normal & even necessary for our health, by our parents, family, friends, relatives, doctors, teachers, clergy & the media in all forms. So, here is some "food" for thought.

It is high time to fully awaken from this cultural trance. In fact, according to the United Nations, the survival of planet Earth depends on it.

As Leonardo da Vinci said, *"The time will come when men such as I will look upon the murder of animals as they now look on the murder of men."* Hopefully, this book will help to bring that time to **now**!

One of my favorite sayings is, *"It is better to light a candle than to curse the darkness."* This book is my attempt to light a candle. It is my hope & prayer that this candle will light your candle & your candle will light other candles until countless candles are lit & we are all illuminated in the lovingkindness of *ahimsa*.

Ahimsa is a Sanskrit word that means to do our best to minimize harm in our thoughts, words & actions.

We are all animals, human & non-human. We virtually all have a similar central nervous system, with a brain, a central cord (or two cords running in parallel) & nerves radiating from the brain & central cord. The only multicellular animals without this are sponges, echinoderms & certain worms.

All mammals, birds, fishes & other vertebrates share the same basic nervous system & neurochemicals, with the attendant perceptions & feelings which are integrated & give rise to the experience of pleasure & pain.

In 2012, the Cambridge Declaration on Consciousness was delivered by a wide spectrum of the world's leading neuroscientists, declaring that non-human animals have the "neurological substrates" to experience emotions & moods.

While it is great to have scientific confirmation, we certainly don't need scientists to tell us that animals have feelings. Anyone who has a companion animal or a modicum of empathy could tell us that!

Through observation & scientific documentation, we can all recognize that human & non-human animals all experience fear, pain, loss & sorrow, as well as joy, love, playfulness & hope.

We all want to enjoy this beautiful planet with our loved ones.
We all have bonds with our family & friends.
We all want to be sovereign & free.

People love their companion animals & consider them to be members of their family. When a beloved pet dies, many people grieve just as if a family member had passed away, & in some cases, even more so.

It is my sincere hope & prayer that the information & inspiration in this book will contribute to an awakening in consciousness that will catalyze a shift from indifference & cruelty to lovingkindness & cooperation.

I believe that people are essentially good at heart & compassionate by nature. When we fully realize the effect that our dietary choices have on every aspect of life, we will be inspired to make more compassionate & sustainable dietary choices that are kind to the animals, to the environment, to human health & wellbeing on all levels.

One of the greatest existential threats that we are facing on planet Earth today is the climate crisis. Many highly respected independent scientists agree that if major changes are not made in this decade, our life on Earth could become uninhabitable. Many top political leaders consider it a leading priority to be addressed at the global level.

Choosing a plant-based diet can help to significantly reduce the climate crisis because, according to a *World Bank* study, about 50% of all greenhouse gas emissions come from animal agriculture. So, by choosing a plant-based diet, we can help reverse one of the greatest threats to the survival of planet Earth. I elaborate on this further in this book, as well as many other profound benefits of choosing a plant-based diet, including preventing future pandemics.

It is possible that pandemics can be prevented because, according to scientists, coronaviruses may be zoonotic, meaning they are transmitted from animals to people. Humans created factory farms, wet markets & small-scale animal exploitation operations, which are breeding grounds for infectious disease agents. Humans cramming animals in crowded cages causes unnatural spikes in harmful toxins & disease factors that can spread from animals to humans.

The toxicity from the agribusiness chemicals & the perverse common practices of animal agriculture perpetuate unnecessary disease & suffering. Wearing face masks, closing down businesses & physically distancing may become commonplace in the world unless animal agriculture operations are shut down. The real *Soulution* is to stop abusing animals & to embrace a plant-based diet.

Our great Creator has graciously provided all the nutrients that we need to be healthy & thrive from the plant kingdom without causing harm to animals or creating breeding grounds for future pandemics.

Additionally, big meat producers are investing millions of dollars in plant-based protein products. Given that nine of the ten largest meat producers in the US have either bought existing plant-based food brands, launched their own, or entered into collaborations with plant-based companies, plant-based food is rapidly going mainstream!

Companies such as Beyond Meat, Tyson Foods, Cargill, Smithfield Foods, Kellogg, Nestle, Hormel Foods, Perdue Farms, ConAgra Brands, Maple Leaf & Impossible Foods are partnering with McDonald's, Subway, Starbucks, Pizza Hut, Burger King, Wendy's, Taco Bell, Domino's Pizza, Dunkin' Donuts & Dairy Queen, helping to facilitate transitioning to a plant-based diet without compromising the tastes & textures to which meat & dairy consumers are accustomed.

Shifting to plant-based nutrition will not only help reverse the climate crisis & prevent future pandemics, but it is *the Soulution* to every major problem that we are facing on planet Earth.

Choosing a plant-based diet will put an end to world hunger because, according to *EarthSave*, it takes 2,500 gallons of water, 12 pounds of grain, 35 pounds of topsoil & the energy equivalent of one gallon of gasoline to produce one pound of feedlot beef.

It requires significantly fewer resources to produce a comparable amount of healthy & delicious plant-based nutrition. According to a report by *Faunalytics*, "Plant-based agriculture grows 512% more pounds of food than animal-based agriculture on 69% of the mass of land that animal-based agriculture uses."

If the US would reduce its consumption of meat, dairy & eggs by just 10%, every one of the 9.1 million people worldwide who die of starvation each year could be fed.

War would also end because when we replace the consciousness of domination & violence with *ahimsa* (nonviolence) & lovingkindness, we can replace war with diplomatic win/win negotiation. We can co-create a peaceful world where we all thrive by giving & receiving our gifts & talents! We all win when we support & collaborate rather than tear down & destroy.

In the pages that follow, I elaborate on how a shift to plant-based nutrition is the individual & global *Soulution* for physical, mental, emotional, spiritual, environmental, cultural & material wellbeing.

Health truly is our greatest wealth! It is very difficult to accomplish anything, whether it be spiritual or material, without good health.

★ Nearly half of the adult population in the US has diabetes or pre-diabetes.

★ Three out of 4 adults in the US are overweight.

★ One in 5 children & adolescents are battling obesity.

★ Illness & food allergies are skyrocketing in our children.

★ The average senior citizen is taking 5 prescription drugs.

★ The rate of Alzheimer's disease is soaring & expected to increase to 35.6 percent by 2025.

★ The top 2 causes of death in the US are heart disease & cancer.

Despite all the media attention given to pandemics, heart disease is still by far, the leading cause of death in developed countries. In fact, cardiovascular disease kills 18 million people each year, which represents 31% of deaths worldwide.

There is indisputable scientific evidence that shows we can significantly lower our risk of all of these health problems, as well as a host of other illnesses, by implementing a plant-based diet. In fact, according to thousands of studies published in peer reviewed medical journals, the single biggest factor for reversing these health problems is the food that we consume.

So, if you care about your health & the health of your loved ones, the animals & the environment upon which all of our lives depend, read on! This book clearly outlines *the Soulution* to reversing every major problem that we face on Earth today!

An ounce of practice is worth more than a ton of theory. By understanding the root cause of all of these problems & by making simple, delicious, nutritious, fun new choices, we all become part of *the Soulution*. Together we can co-create life on Earth to be a healthy & happy paradise for one & all!

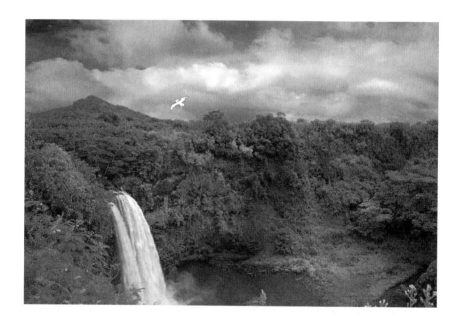

Being a Voice

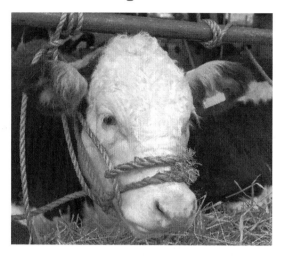

"Never, never be afraid to do what's right, especially if the well-being of a person or animal is at stake. Society's punishments are small compared to the wounds we inflict on our soul when we look the other way."
- Dr. Martin Luther King, Jr.

In this age of over information, why one more book?

Because I want to be a voice for all the unheard & ignored voices.

I want to be a voice for the 72 billion land animals & over a trillion sea creatures who are tortured & killed for meat, fish, dairy & eggs every year.

I want to be a voice for the dairy cows who are forced onto racks & raped through a perverse & painful method of artificial insemination to keep them lactating so they can be exploited as milk machines.

I want to be a voice for both the mother cow & for the baby calf who is ripped away from his or her mother only hours after birth.

I want to be a voice for the anguish in their voices due to being ripped apart.

I want to be a voice for the calves who are chained & caged for veal.

I want to be a voice for the female calves who are forced to live their entire lives confined & tortured to be milk machines like their mothers.

I want to be a voice for their cries of pain as their udders & teats are gouged by metal machines & as they are brutally dehorned, mutilated & forced to stand in their own excrement in hyperconfining stalls, where they cannot even turn around.

I want to be a voice for the hens who are forced to live their entire lives in stacked wire cages with only as much living space as a letter-size sheet of paper.

I want to be a voice for the male baby chicks who are ground up alive or suffocated & thrown in dumpsters.

I want to be a voice for the human mother whose baby is dying in her arms from malnutrition because we are feeding our grains to animals for meat & dairy instead of to children who are starving to death.

I want to be a voice for all those who are suffering from water shortages because it takes 2,500 gallons of water to produce one pound of meat & 1,000 gallons of water to produce a gallon of milk, whereas it takes only 250 gallons of water to produce one pound of plant food.

I want to be a voice for our forests—the lungs of our planet—that are being cut down at an alarming rate to graze cows & grow crops to feed animals being used for meat.

I want to be a voice for the 200 species that become extinct on Earth every day due to animal agriculture's deforestation, loss of habit & pollution.

I want to be a voice for the rivers, lakes, streams & oceans that are being polluted by the toxic waste & excrement from factory farms.

I want to be a voice for those living in poor communities near these factory farms, forced to breathe the hideous stench & drink the polluted water caused by these concentration camps for animals.

I want to be a voice for the slaughterhouse workers who are traumatized by murdering animals all day & then take out their frustrations through domestic violence, addiction & crime.

I want to be a voice for human health because heart disease, cancer, obesity, diabetes & a host of other health issues can all be reversed through a low-fat vegan diet, along with other healthy lifestyle choices.

I want to be a voice for everyone who is suffering as a result of global pandemics. Confining, abusing & killing animals on mass scales creates breeding grounds for infectious disease agents that transmit to humans.

I want to be a voice for *the Soulution* to the climate crisis, which is one of the greatest existential threats to the survival of life on Earth.

I want to be a voice for reversing antibiotic resistance that is caused by the fact that 80% of our antibiotics are forced on animals used for meat.

I want to be a voice to alleviate & eliminate the suffering of all social injustices that arise from the consciousness of domination & violence.

I want to be a compassionate, effective, strong, far-reaching voice for lovingkindness & *ahimsa* (non-violence).

I want to take my last breath knowing that I used my mind, body, heart, soul, intelligence, compassion & all of the faculties & resources given to me by our great Creator to be a voice; to take a stand for what is right & to help awaken the masses from this cultural trance so that together, we can replace unconscious cruelty with lovingkindness to all!

I want to be a voice because, as Emerson said,
"To know even one life has breathed easier because you have lived. This is to have succeeded."

May we all succeed by going vegan!

Definitions

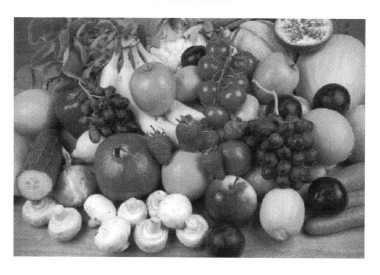

"The beginning of wisdom is the definition of terms."
- Socrates

There is a lot of confusion about the differences between a vegetarian diet & a vegan diet. Contrary to popular belief, there is no such thing as a fish-eating or chicken-eating vegetarian. By definition, vegetarians do not eat any type of flesh. Here are some common definitions ~

Vegetarian, also called lacto-ovo vegetarian
Eats no meat of any kind, including fish or chicken. Eats eggs & dairy products.

Lacto-vegetarian
Eats no meat of any kind, including fish or chicken. Eats dairy products, but not eggs.

Ovo-vegetarian
Eats no meat of any kind, including fish or chicken. Eats eggs, but not dairy products.

Vegan
Eats no meat of any kind & eats no products that come from animals, including eggs & dairy.

Many vegans also exclude honey from their diets & take a stand against beekeeping practices that harm bee health. After all, one out of every three bites of food that we eat relies on pollinators. Where would we be without them?

There are, however, some devoted vegans & vegan advocates who feel that bees can thrive with compassionate organic beekeepers. (I elaborate on this further in the *To Bee or Not to Bee* section.)

Raw foodist
Raw foodists eat only uncooked foods. They generally eat fresh fruits, vegetables, seeds, nuts & sprouts. They believe that foods lose their enzymes when they are cooked &/or processed. Raw foodists are not necessarily vegan or even vegetarian. Some raw foodists eat raw fish or other raw meat, although this is the exception rather than the rule.

Ahimsa
Ahimsa is a Sanskrit word that means nonviolence. It means to do our best not to cause harm in our thoughts, words & actions. To me, the essence of nonviolence is lovingkindness. With lovingkindness, we go beyond not causing harm & do our best to be a benevolent, beneficial presence. This is the foundation for the *Lovingkindness Diet & Lifestyle*.

Veganism is more than a diet. It is a state of consciousness based on *ahimsa*. In addition to not eating animal products, many vegans do not use any products that come from animals such as leather, fur, wool, silk, down, non-vegan cosmetics, non-vegan household products & any other products that come from abusing animals.

Many vegans work to put an end to exploiting & abusing animals for "entertainment," such as elephants, wild animals in circuses, zoos, dolphins & whales in captivity, horse racing, greyhound racing, sled dog racing, rodeos, bullfights & organized animal fighting.

Many vegans also work to put an end to cruel & unnecessary animal testing.

So, when defining *veganism*, I want to emphasize that it is far more than a diet; it is a lifestyle based on *ahimsa* (nonviolence). It is a mindset that guides & drives our choices to do our best to replace cruelty & injustices, in any form, with kind treatment toward one & all.

> ***"Kindness is the highest form of wisdom."***
> - The Talmud

Supercharge Your Wellbeing on All Levels with the Lovingkindness Diet & Lifestyle

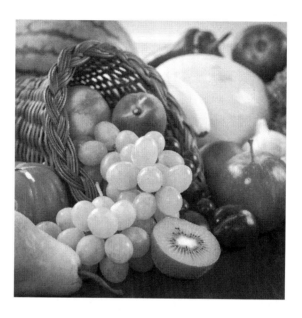

"Kindness is the sunshine in which virtue grows."
- Robert Green Ingersoll

I wrote in my last book, *Feel Good Now: How to Feel Your Best & Have Your Best to Give*, that the goal of all goals is to feel good. What we eat has a huge impact on how we feel!

If you want to feel your best & have your best to give, I highly recommend supercharging your wellbeing with *The Lovingkindness Diet & Lifestyle*.

Why? Because what goes around comes around!

If you choose food that is kind to the animals, to the environment & to your own health, kindness is what will return to you on all levels!

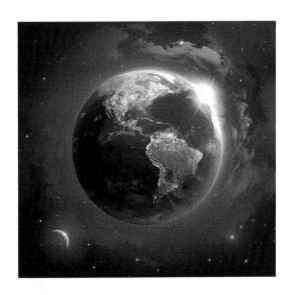

Problems existing on Earth today include droughts, fires, deforestation, climate destabilization, pollution, depletion of farmlands, ocean devastation, energy shortages, world hunger, disease, animal suffering, domestic & international violence, global pandemics & so much more.

Few people are aware that what we eat is directly related to the crises that we face on Earth today.

The SAD—meaning the Standard America Diet, which consists of meat, fowl, fish, dairy & eggs—is one of the major causes of all of these problems.

It is also one of the major causes of heart disease, cancer, obesity, diabetes, autoimmune diseases, infectious diseases & a multitude of other health issues.

By choosing the GLAD vegan diet—which consists of fruit, vegetables, grains, legumes, nuts, seeds & sprouts—all of these problems can be reversed!

GLAD, in this context, stands for the *Global Loving Ahimsa Diet*. (*Ahimsa* is a Sanskrit word meaning nonviolence.) It is high time to connect the dots & make some new choices for the benefit of one & all! So, here are my *10 Compelling Reasons to Choose a Plant-based Diet!*

10 Compelling Reasons to Choose the Lovingkindness Diet & Lifestyle
Connecting the Dots

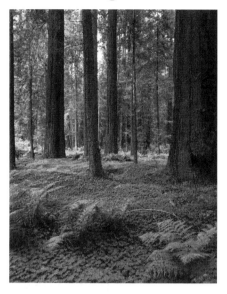

"A single act of kindness throws out roots in all directions & the roots spring up & make new trees."
- Amelia Earhart

- ★ Animal Welfare
- ★ Eliminate World Hunger & Starvation
- ★ Reverse Water Shortage
- ★ Reverse Deforestation
- ★ Reverse the Climate Crisis
- ★ Reverse Pollution
- ★ Increase Energy ~ Individual & Global
- ★ Improve Health & Prevent Future Pandemics
- ★ Eliminate Modern Day Slavery & Put an End to War
- ★ It is the Right Thing to Do!

1) Animal Welfare

"The greatness of a nation & its moral progress can be judged by the way its animals are treated."
- Mahatma Gandhi

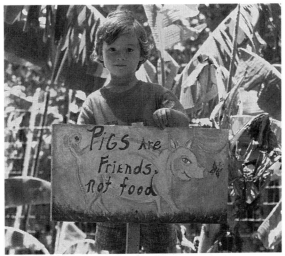

My precious friend, Koa Le'amohala
at Leilani Farm Sanctuary, Maui, HI

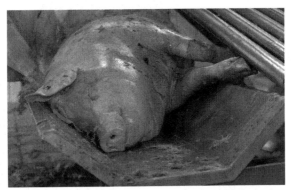

Although most people are more familiar with their pets—such as cats, dogs & parakeets—than they are with cows, pigs, chickens & fishes, animals used for food are as intelligent & able to feel pain as the animals with whom we share our homes.

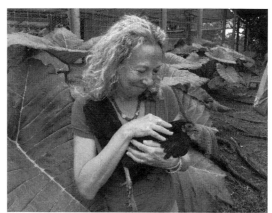

My precious sister, Jiya Kowarsky,
at Leilani Farm Sanctuary, Maui HI

★ Pigs can learn to play video games & chickens are so smart that their intelligence has been compared by scientists to that of monkeys.

★ More than 72 billion land animals & over a trillion marine animals are killed every year for meat, seafood, dairy & eggs!

★ 99% of these animals are kept in factory farms, which are concentration camps for animals & cause horrific suffering to these living beings.

★ These factory farms are disease-ridden to the extent that animals are fed, injected & sprayed with antibiotics, insecticides & other toxic substances just to keep them alive.

★ Animals are injected with hormones to make them grow both fatter & faster.

★ Dairy cows are injected with hormones to make them produce more milk.

* According to PETA, pigs in these factory farms, which is where 99% of pork comes from, never get to take a breath of fresh air or nurture their young.

* Dairy cows are in such terrible shape that they frequently collapse during their ride to the slaughterhouse, where they are prodded or dragged off the trucks, often resulting in their bones breaking as they hit the ground.

* Chickens & turkeys are crammed into crowded sheds with tens of thousands of other birds where disease, being smothered & having heart attacks are common occurrences.

* When animals are taken to slaughterhouses, they see, smell & feel the terror. Just as we would anticipate something terrible is about to happen, so do these animals. They show signs of stress, such as increases in cortisol, high-pitched vocalizations, panting, etc.

* Since the meat, dairy & egg industries are based on supply & demand, by purchasing & eating these products, we are the prime causal agent of this horrific cruelty.

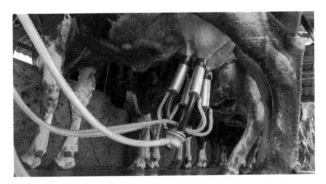

* We are also ingesting these toxic substances, plus the biochemistry of misery & terror that is aroused by the mistreatment & slaughter of these living beings.

★ All vertebrates can & do feel pain, just as we do. Is any meat, dairy product or egg worth causing this unnecessary suffering to these precious animals?

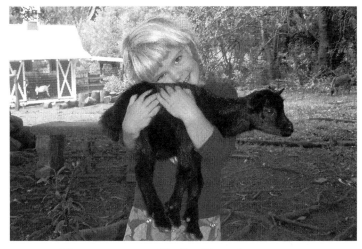

Photo courtesy of LeilaniFarmSanctuary.org

★ Let's remember to treat others as we would like to be treated. What goes around comes around!

★ Every vegan saves about 200 animals each year & thousands over a lifetime. Vegan advocates help to save even more animals.

★ "When meat eaters look at a cow they see a hamburger. When vegans look at a hamburger they see a cow."

★ Choosing vegan foods over meat, eggs & dairy products is an effective way to prevent suffering & eliminate animal abuse.

★ With every bite we take, we are either voting for cruelty or lovingkindness toward the animals, the environment & our own health. So, let's choose wisely!

2) Eliminate World Hunger & Starvation

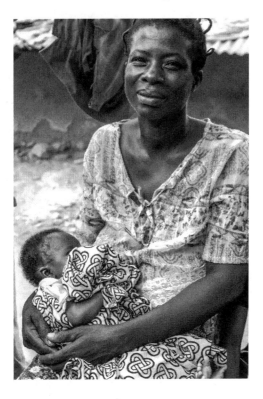

"What does love look like? It has the hands to help others. It has the feet to hasten to the poor and needy. It has eyes to see misery and want. It has the ears to hear the sighs and sorrows of men. That is what love looks like."
- St. Augustine

★ It takes up to 16 pounds of grain to produce just one pound of meat. All that plant food can be used much more efficiently if it is fed directly to people.

★ One acre of farmland can feed 20 times as many people who are eating a GLAD vegan diet than those eating a SAD diet.

★ According to a summary by *Faunalytics*, plant-based agriculture generates around 1.5 trillion more pounds of food than animal agriculture & it does so more efficiently.

★ The *Faunalytics* report concludes that "plant-based agriculture grows 512% more pounds of food than animal-based agriculture on 69% of the mass of land that animal-based agriculture uses."

★ If the USA would reduce its consumption of the SAD diet by just 10%, every one of the 9.1 million people worldwide who die of starvation each year could be fed.

★ Is any meat, dairy product, or egg worth not eliminating starvation worldwide? Help end world hunger by choosing the GLAD vegan diet & we will all be glad!

3) Reverse Water Shortage

"When the well is dry, we know the worth of water."
- Benjamin Franklin

By going vegan, we can transform this ~

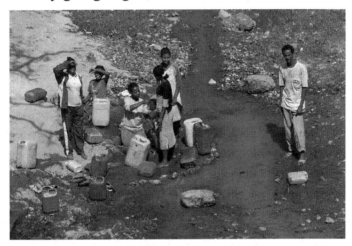

to this, for everybody!

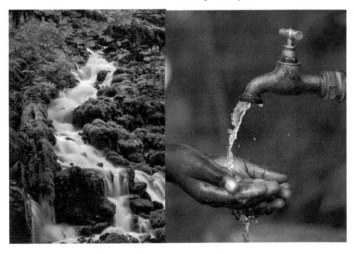

★ Over 40% of the world is facing a water shortage.

★ The meat industry alone uses over 50% of all water in the United States.

★ It takes over 2,500 gallons of water to produce one pound of meat, whereas it takes about 250 gallons of water to produce one pound of grain.

★ Every time we eat a GLAD vegan meal instead of a SAD meal, we are saving hundreds of gallons of water.

★ According to Water Calculator, someone following a vegan diet has half the total water footprint as a meat-eater.

4) Reverse Deforestation

"Forests are the world's air-conditioning system—the lungs of our planet—and we are on the verge of switching it off."
- Prince Charles

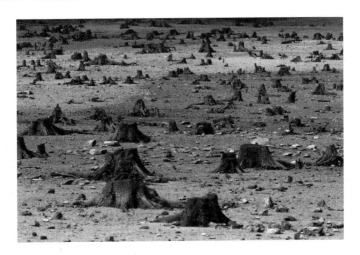

★ Animal agriculture accounts for more than 80% of deforestation.

★ Fifty million acres of Earth's forests vanish in a single week.

★ A piece of rainforest the size of ten city blocks disappears every minute.

★ Animal agriculture is responsible for 91% of the destruction of the Amazon Forest.

★ Over 3 million acres of US forests have been cleared for cropland to produce the SAD diet.

★ The cost of mass-producing cattle, poultry, pigs, sheep & fish is intensifying the destruction of forests on which our planet's life-cycles depend.

* Oxford University researchers completed the most comprehensive analysis of farming's impact on the planet. They looked at data from approximately 40,000 farms in 119 countries & found that beef production requires 36 times more land than plant-based protein like peas. The researchers stated that if everyone were to go vegan, global farmland use would drop by 75 %, freeing up a landmass the size of Australia, China, the E.U. & the USA combined.

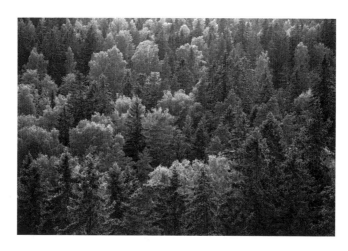

* Trees absorb carbon dioxide & give off oxygen. When trees are gone, life, as we know it on Earth, will also be gone.

* According to the *UN Environment Programme*, 200 species become extinct every day due to deforestation, loss of habitat & pollution. Scientists state that this is unlike anything seen since the dinosaurs disappeared 65 million years ago.

* By choosing the GLAD vegan diet rather than the SAD diet, we can reverse the destruction of forests, reduce global warming & preserve life on Earth for future generations.

5) Reverse Global Warming & The Climate Crisis

"Adults keep saying we owe it to the young people, to give them hope, but I don't want your hope. I don't want you to be hopeful. I want you to panic. I want you to feel the fear I feel every day. I want you to act. I want you to act as you would in a crisis. I want you to act as if the house is on fire, because it is."
- Greta Thunberg, 16-year-old Environmental Activist

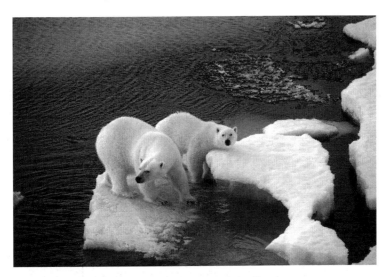

The climate crisis is one of humankind's greatest environmental threats. According to the United Nations, climate change is affecting every continent, impacting agriculture, human health, ecosystems, water supplies, people's livelihoods & every aspect of life on Earth.

★ Animal agriculture is one of the major generators of greenhouse gas emissions, which worsens climate change.

★ The UNEP (United Nations Environmental Programme) has named meat "the world's most urgent problem," saying that, "Our use of animals as a food-production technology has brought us to the verge of catastrophe."

* The SAD diet contributes to the greenhouse effect through the release of carbon dioxide, methane gas & nitrous oxide into the atmosphere.

* Carbon dioxide, methane, & nitrous oxide are all powerful greenhouse gases, & together, they cause the vast majority of climate destabilization.

Carbon Dioxide

* Burning fossil fuels, such as oil & gasoline, release carbon dioxide. According to PETA, it takes about 11 times as much fossil fuel to produce a calorie of animal protein as it does to produce a calorie of grain protein & considerably more carbon dioxide is released. It is more climate efficient to produce protein from vegetable sources than from animal sources.

* Deforestation, for grazing cows & for growing crops to feed animals for meat & dairy products, increases carbon dioxide rapidly, while destroying trees, which absorb the carbon dioxide.

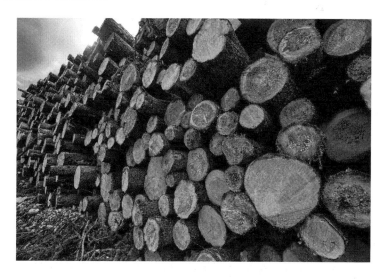

Methane

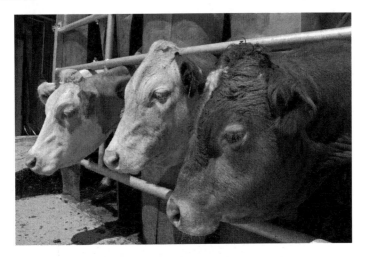

* The billions of imprisoned animals who are confined on both factory farms as well as free-range operations, produce enormous amounts of methane. Ruminants, such as cows, sheep & goats, produce methane gas as part of their digestive process.

* Methane is also emitted from thousands of acres of cesspools filled with the feces excreted by pigs, cows & other animals in factory farms.

* The United States Environmental Protection Agency has shown that animal agriculture is the largest source of global methane gas emissions & that, over a 20 year period, methane is 84 times more efficient than carbon dioxide at trapping heat in our atmosphere, contributing to global warming.
https://www.edf.org/climate/methane-other-important-greenhouse-gas

Nitrous Oxide

★ Nitrous oxide, which is released from synthetic fertilizer & manure in factory farms, is about 300 times more potent as a greenhouse gas than carbon dioxide.

★ According to the U.N., the meat, dairy & egg industries account for 65% of worldwide nitrous oxide emissions.

★ It is energy-intensive to grow massive amounts of grain & water to feed animals raised for meat, as well as to slaughter, process, transport, refrigerate & store their flesh & secretions.

★ Many people are trying to combat the climate crisis by driving more fuel-efficient cars & using energy-saving light bulbs. While these measures are a step in the right direction, they simply are not enough to reverse the climate crisis.

★ A University of Chicago study showed that you can reduce your carbon footprint more effectively by going vegan than by switching from a conventional car to a hybrid.

★ Producing half a pound of beef generates the same amount of emissions as driving a car 9.8 miles. Producing half a pound of potatoes is equal to driving a car 0.17 miles.

★ According to the United Nations Food & Agriculture Organization official study, animal agriculture generates 18% of the world's greenhouse gas emissions, which is even more than the emissions generated by all forms of transportation!

* According to a study commissioned by the World Bank, this 18% figure is a severe underestimate & should actually be about 51%.

* A study at Oxford University, published in the journal *Climatic Change*, shows that meat-eaters are responsible for almost twice as many dietary greenhouse gas emissions per day as vegetarians & about two & a half as many as vegans.

* Researchers with Loma Linda University in California found that vegans have the smallest carbon footprint, generating a 41.7% smaller volume of greenhouse gasses than meat-eaters do.

* The U.N. states that a global shift toward plant-based food is vital, if we are to combat the detrimental effects of climate change.

* Did you know that dog food accounts for 30% of America's meat carbon footprint? A study released by UCLA calculated that the meat-based food eaten by Americans' dogs & cats generates the equivalent of 64 million tons of carbon dioxide per year, which has about the same climate impact as a year's worth of driving from 13.6 million cars.

* Our dogs need protein, not meat. Many people believe dogs are carnivores. In reality, dogs can digest protein from multiple sources because dogs are omnivores. Dogs require 10 essential amino acids to thrive & all 10 can be found in plants.

★ For conscientious dog guardians, *Wild Earth*, *Evolution* & *V-Dog*, among others, deliver responsible dog food to our doorsteps. There are high-protein, high-fiber dog foods that are meat-free, made with ingredients that nourish our companion animals, our planet & our desire to do the right thing.

★ If we care about protecting the environment & reversing the climate crisis, the most powerful step we can take as individuals is to stop eating meat, eggs & dairy products for ourselves & for our companion animals (pets).

★ Killing animals is killing our planet. Eating plant-based food rather than animal-based food is the best way to reduce our carbon footprint. So, if you think you are an environmentalist & you are not a vegan, think again!

★ When we eat the GLAD vegan diet, instead of the SAD diet, we significantly reduce global warming & contribute to the healing of our climate & our Earth, not only for ourselves but for future generations.

6) Reverse Pollution

"Be part of the Soulution, not the pollution!"
- Meenakshi Angel Honig

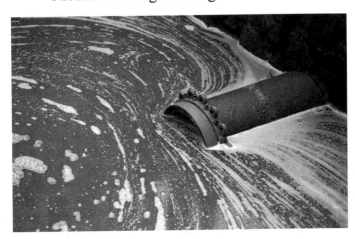

★ 99% of animals raised & killed for the SAD diet are kept in factory farms, which are hyper-confining concentration camps for animals.

★ These imprisoned animals produce over 20 times more excrement than the entire human population!

★ Because these animals are injected, fed & sprayed with pesticides & antibiotics, the water is filled with toxic chemicals. This toxic water is then dumped, untreated, into lakes & rivers, ending up in oceans & aquifers.

★ According to the *National Water Quality Inventory*, 70% of lakes, reservoirs & ponds; 78% of bays & estuaries; & 55% of rivers & streams assessed in the USA are impaired by pollution & do not meet minimum water quality standards.

★ 80% of all organic water pollution in the US is attributable to the SAD diet.

★ The pesticides, herbicides & fertilizers used on feed crops enter & pollute waterways & aquifers. Factory farm runoff & livestock grazing are major contributors to river, lake & ocean pollution.

★ According to the documentary film *Cowspiracy*, animal agriculture creates 70% to 90% of freshwater pollution in western countries.

★ A 2018 report published in the journal *Current Biology* discovered that 87% of the world's oceans are dying. Half of the plastic found in the ocean comes from fishing nets.

★ By choosing the GLAD vegan diet over the SAD, meat, fish, dairy & eggs diet, we can reverse pollution & restore clean flowing water to our precious mother Earth for the benefit of one & all!

7) Increase Energy ~ Individual & Global

"When the winds of change blow, some people build walls, others build windmills."
- Chinese Proverb

Animal protein production requires about 11 times as much fossil fuel energy to produce as a comparable amount of plant protein.

The SAD diet accounts for over 33% of all fossil fuels used in the US.

The GLAD vegan diet would not only cut our oil imports but could increase the supply of renewable energy, such as wood & hydroelectric, by 120%.

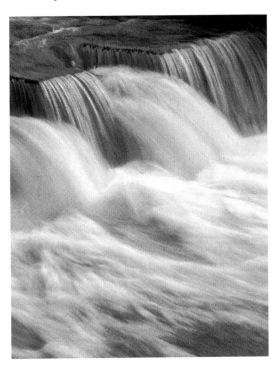

* By choosing the GLAD diet, we also have more internal energy because we are not polluting our body temples & draining our vital life-force energy with the biochemistry of misery, toxins & saturated fat that come with the SAD diet.

* Meat, dairy, & eggs require more energy to digest than plant-based products. By going vegan, you have more energy available to fuel your mind & body & attune to Spirit!

* Nikola Tesla said, *"So we find that the three possible solutions of the great problem of increasing human energy are answered by the three words: food, peace, work."*

* Therefore, let's eat plant-based ***food*** that promotes ***peace*** on all levels & ***work*** for that outcome so that we can be the ***Soulution*** in creating a world that works for all of us.

8) Improve Health & Prevent Future Pandemics

"Every human being is the author of his own health or disease."
- Buddha

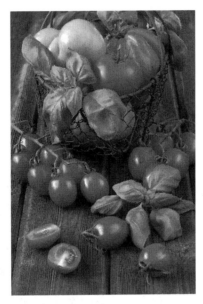

★ Heart disease & cancer are the two leading causes of death in the USA.

★ Dietary cholesterol & saturated fats are major causes of heart attacks.

★ The SAD diet is high in cholesterol & saturated fats, whereas the GLAD vegan diet is free of cholesterol & low in fat.

★ The risk of heart attacks & cancer is significantly reduced for those eating a GLAD vegan diet.

★ The cholesterol & saturated animal fat found in meat, eggs & dairy products clog the arteries to the heart.

* Over time, this impedes the blood flow to other vital organs, which also contributes to sexual malfunction.

* Processed meat is often contaminated with feces, blood & other bodily fluids, making animal products one of the top sources of food poisoning in the United States. This results in diarrhea, cramping, abdominal pain & fever.

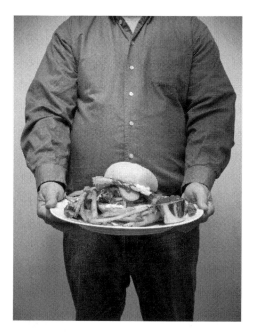

A man said to the waiter, "I'll have the double deluxe bacon cheeseburger." The waiter replied, "Would you like chemotherapy with that?"

* Eating animals that have been given hormones to speed growth, which is a common practice in the meat industry, means those hormones go into our bodies.

* Not only does this disrupt the natural balance of our hormones, but some of the hormones given to animals have been shown to cause tumor growth in humans.

* The breast milk of mothers eating a SAD diet is becoming increasingly contaminated with toxins, while the breast milk of mothers eating the GLAD vegan diet contains only 1 to 2% of this contamination.

* According to Dr. Neal Bernard, founding president of the Physicians Committee for Responsible Medicine, 80% of all antibiotics go to factory farms to be used on animals. Because the bacteria are exposed to antibiotics, they develop resistance to them, which is destroying antibiotics for doctors to prescribe to humans for illnesses such as pneumonia, urinary tract infections & so forth. Doctors have been speaking out against this for a long time, but big Pharma seems to care more about big profits than human health.

* These antibiotics also go into our body temple when we eat the flesh & secretions of these animals. Please keep in mind that 99% of meat, dairy & eggs in the United States come from factory farms, where this is a routine practice.

* Vegans are, on average, up to twenty pounds lighter than meat-eaters. Going vegan is a healthy way to keep excess fat off for good while increasing your energy.

* Being an agent of cruelty—ingesting the biochemistry of terror, toxic chemicals & the fat contained in the SAD diet— contributes to allergies, depression, anxiety, obesity, high blood pressure, arthritis, aches & pains, poor sleep, sexual malfunction & a host of other health issues.

* In contrast, ingesting the GLAD vegan diet contributes to good health, happiness, mental clarity, vitality, ideal weight, sound sleep & overall wellbeing!

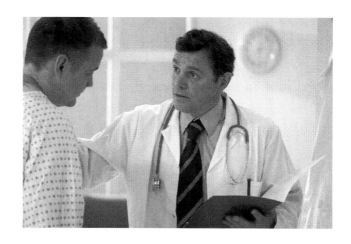

A heart surgeon said to his patient, "*So, you have two options. We could perform triple bypass surgery, where we take a vein out of your thigh & cut open your chest so we can sew the vein onto your coronary artery. This costs over $100,000 & you will be restricted to bed rest for at least two months. Or, option number two is: We could put you on a vegan diet. The patient responded, "A vegan diet? Gee Doc, that sounds pretty radical."*
- Based on a quote from Dr. Caldwell Esselstyn

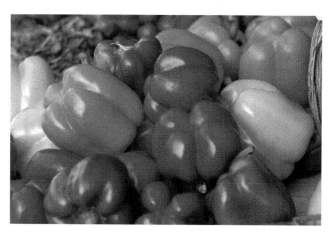

★ The GLAD vegan diet is a no-cholesterol, low-fat, high-fiber diet consisting of fruits, vegetables, grains, beans, nuts & seeds, which supply ample protein for our human bodies.

★ The SAD diet of meat, dairy & eggs provides more protein than the human body needs.

★ Our bodies take calcium from our bones in an attempt to neutralize the acid load caused by this excess protein, contributing to such diseases as osteoporosis & kidney failure.

★ A study published in *Topics in Integrative Health Care* found fruit & vegetables are all you need for healthy bones & that osteoporosis, the condition that weakens bones & makes them brittle, is actually more prevalent in the developed countries where more dairy products are consumed.

★ If you want quality calcium that will *"do your body good,"* replace dairy products with greens because 100 grams of kale contain more calcium than 100 grams of milk, without the toxins, fat & misery contained in milk.

★ The GLAD vegan diet improves your gut health which makes you feel better both mentally & physically. Tiny bacteria play an important role in everything from your digestion to your immune system & mood.

★ According to a 2014 review published in the journal *Nutrients*, when compared to meat-eating & even vegetarian diets, vegans' gut profiles are top-notch with less disease-causing organisms & more protective species of bacteria, as well as lower levels of inflammation.

★ The GLAD diet also helps you breathe better! According to *earthis.com*, a group study of participants with serious asthma issues, who had been taking medication for around 12 years, ate a vegan diet for a year. Nearly all of them no longer had any asthma symptoms & were able to either get rid of or reduce their medications.

★ Due to our social indoctrination, people often ask vegans, *"Where do you get your protein?"* It would be impossible not to get enough protein if you are eating a whole food plant-based diet, provided you are eating enough food, such as a standard 2000-calorie-per-day diet.

Where do you get your protein?

No Meat? No Problem!
Protein is in everything, even fruit.

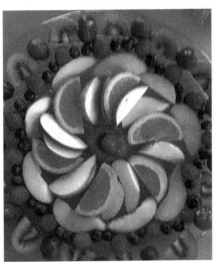

Photo by Meenakshi Angel Honig

	Protein	Fiber
Apples	0.5 g	4.6 g
Bananas	1.2 g	2.9 g
Oranges	1.9 g	4.5 g
Rice	2.1 g	0.3 g
Pasta	4.2 g	2.3 g
Chickpeas	5.3 g	7.6 g
Kidney Beans	6.7 g	4.4 g
Peas	6.7 g	6.3 g
Lentils	7.0 g	4.4 g
Broccoli	8.3 g	7.6 g
Tofu	11.7 g	1.3 g
Spinach	12.4 g	9.6 g

(Data is based on 100 kcals per food. Source: www.veganstreet.com)

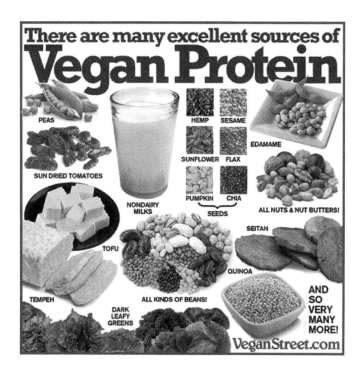

* Peanut butter & jelly on whole wheat bread ~ 14g protein
  McDonald's hamburger ~ 13g protein
  Protein certainly doesn't have to come from tortured animals!

* Here are some plant-based foods that are packed with protein ~ pumpkin seeds, asparagus, cauliflower, mung bean sprouts, almonds, spinach, broccoli, quinoa & peanuts.

* Daily protein requirements are 56 grams for men & 46 grams for women.

* In the western world, most people get 2 to 3 times more protein than they actually need. Plant protein comes with plenty of vitamins & minerals & without cholesterol. An excess of animal protein has been linked to cancer growth. (*The China Study*)

★ *"The beef industry has contributed to more American deaths than all the wars of this century, all natural disasters & all automobile accidents combined. If beef is your idea of 'real food for real people' you'd better live real close to a real good hospital."*
- Neal D. Barnard. M.D.

★ The GLAD diet makes you feel glad! In a study from the *American Journal of Health Promotion*, researchers found those who switched over to a plant-based diet had improvements in their symptoms of depression & anxiety, making them feel happier & more at ease.

★ Experts have stated that even with its 99.6% survival rate, COVID-19 severely affected billions of people in 219 countries & territories. The impact of fear, illness, lockdowns, isolation, closing businesses & a lack of healthy diet, exercise & other unhealthy choices, all add up to a massive toll on physical, mental, emotional & economic health.

★ Hmmm, fear, lockdowns, isolation, lack of healthy diet & exercise, etc., isn't this the way that animals are treated in animal agriculture operations? Did humanity really think that we could mercilessly hyper-confine, torture & murder animals, pillage & poison our precious mother Earth & not have any consequences?

★ Pandemics are a golden opportunity for a huge wake up call.

★ The good news is that we can help to prevent future pandemics!

★ Animal agriculture operations are breeding grounds for zoonotic infectious diseases. By shutting them down & choosing plant-based foods, we can help to avoid future outbreaks. I elaborate on this further in the upcoming section on *How to Prevent Future Pandemics*.

★ Health is our greatest wealth! Without it, it is difficult to achieve anything, whether it be spiritual or material. What we ingest has a huge effect on our health & wellbeing, both individually & globally.

★ You have been entrusted to be the steward of your body temple. Out of respect & love for your Creator, for yourself, for your family, for your friends, for everyone who counts on you, for your community & for the world, isn't it worth it to make the healthiest dietary choices?

★ Plant Food: Better for your health, the animals & our planet.

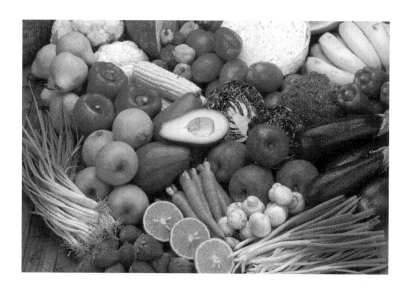

9) Eliminate Modern Day Slavery & Put an End to War

"Those who deny freedom to others, deserve it not for themselves."
- Abraham Lincoln

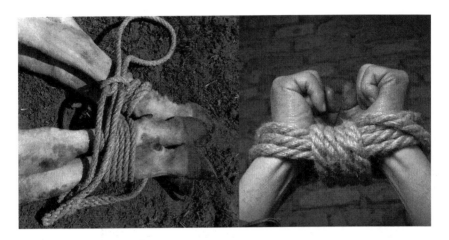

★ Few people realize the connection between animal slavery & human slavery.

★ History changed its course in western Asia about 11,000 years ago when people began exploiting animals, such as goats, sheep & cattle, for their meat, milk, hides & labor.

★ Up until that time, there had been a kinship between human animals & non-human animals.

★ We are by nature kind & compassionate. So, in order for these pre-historic herdsman & farmers to start castrating, hobbling, branding & imprisoning animals to control their mobility, diet, growth & reproductive lives, they had to shut down their innate sensitivity & override their true nature.

* To disconnect themselves emotionally from the cruelty that they were inflicting on animals, they adopted mechanisms such as detachment, rationalization, denial & the use of euphemisms.

* Once this cruel mentality set in & became the new norm, it was not a big jump to inflict this cruelty onto people.

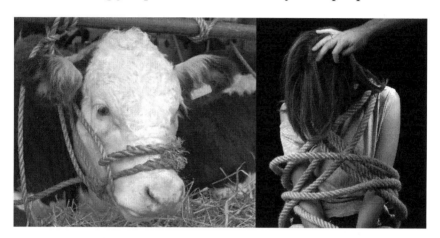

* This mentality of domination & violence paved the way for domestic violence, slavery & war.

* A chattel slave is an enslaved person who is owned forever & whose children & children's children are automatically enslaved. Chattel slaves are individuals treated as mere property, to be bought & sold. The mentality of chattel slavery is the same mentality as cattle slavery.

* Dr. Martin Luther King said, *"A threat to justice anywhere is a threat to justice everywhere."*

* There are more slaves on Earth today than any other time in human history.

* Modern slavery is a multibillion-dollar industry, with just the forced labor aspect generating $150 billion each year. The Global Slavery Index (2018) estimated that roughly 40.3 million individuals are currently caught in modern slavery, with 71% of those being female & one in four being children.

* Modern Day slavery includes ~

    * Child Sex Trafficking
    * Forced Child Marriages
    * Forced Labor
    * Bonded Labor or Debt Bondage
    * Domestic Servitude
    * Forced Child Labor
    * Organ removal
    * Unlawful Recruitment & Use of Child Soldiers

* As Tolstoy said, *"As long as there are slaughterhouses there will be battlegrounds."*

* The consciousness of domination & violence that led to animal slavery, led to human slavery & war. It is this consciousness that is root cause of all of these problems.

* *"The function of freedom is to free someone else."*
  - Toni Morrison

* By replacing the consciousness of violence with the consciousness of *ahimsa*, (nonviolence), backed up by congruent compassionate action, all of these problems can be ameliorated. The violence of war can be replaced with diplomatic negotiation & creative win-win *Soulutions*!

* As Dr. Martin Luther King, Jr., said, *"No one is free until we are all free."*

10) It is the Right Thing to Do!

"On some positions cowardice asks the question, is it safe? Expediency asks the question, is it politic? Vanity asks the question, is it popular? But conscience asks the question, is it right? And there comes a time when one must take a position that is neither safe, nor politic, nor popular but he must take it because conscience tells him it is right."
 - Dr. Martin Luther King Jr.

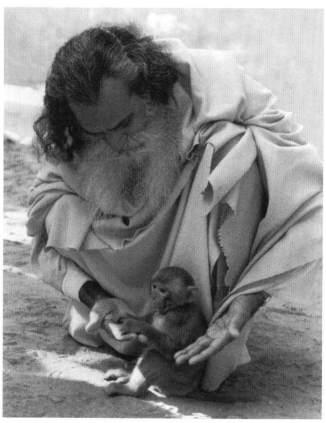

Photo courtesy of Yogaville.org

★ If you ask people if it is morally correct to cause unnecessary suffering to animals, the vast majority will say, "No."

* So, how is it possible that we live in a world where it is considered OK to torture & kill more than 72 billion land animals & over a trillion marine animals per year? Let's wake up from this cultural trance & go vegan!

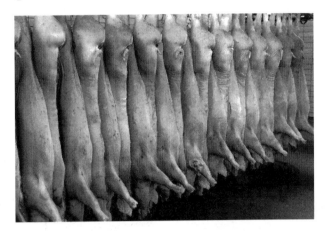

* Since it is based on supply & demand, if we stop buying it, the meat, dairy & egg industries will stop supplying it. It is that simple!

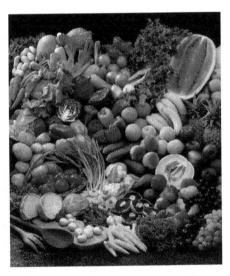

* The food that is best for us is also best for the other forms of life on Earth & for the life support systems upon which we all depend.

* Ingesting the biochemistry of terror & misery from the SAD (Standard American Diet) contributes to domestic violence, modern day slavery & war.

* Ingesting plant-based nutrition that is kind to animals, the environment & human health contributes to personal & global peace & wellbeing.

* The SAD is a major cause of all of the crises that we are facing on planet Earth today. Choosing the GLAD vegan diet reverses all of these problems.

* So, rather than contributing to the problem, why not activate our Soul-force & be part of *the Soulution* by going vegan?

"Nothing will benefit human health & increase the chances for survival of life on earth as much as the evolution to a vegetarian diet."
- Albert Einstein.

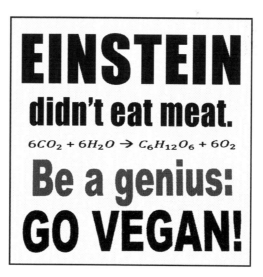

The Vital Importance of Transitioning from Vegetarian to Vegan

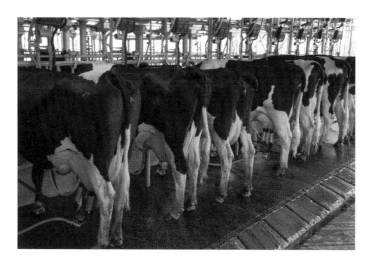

"You may choose to look the other way, but you can never say again that you didn't know."
- William Wilberforce

For those of you who think that being a vegetarian is enough & that it is not necessary to become a vegan, meaning eliminating dairy & eggs from your dietary choices, please consider this carefully ~

★ The dairy & egg industries are two of the cruelest aspects of the meat industry.

★ 99% of dairy in the United States comes from cows in factory farms where they are routinely confined, brutally dehorned, chained, & raped through a painful & perverse process of artificial insemination, milked with electric machines that are painful, & have their newborn calves ripped away from them within hours after birth.

★ After they endure this torture for about four to five years, they are spent & sent to be slaughtered for beef. The natural average lifespan of a cow is 20 - 25 years.

★ So, if you eat dairy products, your voting dollar is paying people to abuse & torture cows & goats. Please pause for a moment; think about that, take it to heart, & seriously consider replacing dairy products with the countless delicious & nutritious substitutes that are so readily available today.

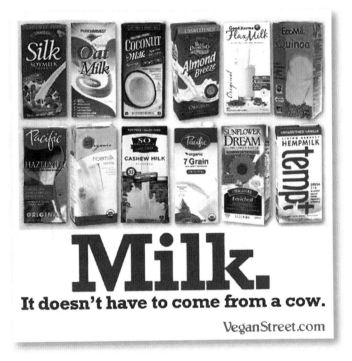

Milk ~ It doesn't have to come from a cow or goat.

As *PETA* says, *"Not your mom, not your milk!"*

Some delicious & nutrient-rich plant milks are ~

* Almond milk
* Coconut milk
* Rice milk
* Soy milk
* Oat milk
* Cashew milk
* Macadamia nut milk
* Hemp milk
* Quinoa milk
* Peanut milk
* Pea milk

Plant milks can also be made from ~

* Barley
* Fonio
* Maize
* Millet
* Sorghum
* Teff
* Triticale
* Spelt
* Wheat

* For all you cheese lovers out there, with so many new plant-based cheeses coming on the market today, which taste better & are free of the toxic effects from dairy cheese, it makes this transition a no brainer.

★ In fact, many cheese lovers have reported that the vegan cheddar, pepper jack, European cultured vegan butter, & organic cultured cream cheese produced by Miyoko's Creamery— *"The Official Cheese of OMGs ~ You Won't Believe It's Made from Plants"*—are their all-time favorite cheeses!

★ These products, along with so many other vegan milk & cheese products, make it so easy to be part of *the Soulution!*

★ Here is a list from *vegan.com* to support you in making an easy & delicious transition ~

Vegan Cheese Brands (USA & Canada)

★ Daiya Foods ~ Shreds, Slices, Blocks & Cream Cheese

★ Dr. Cow ~ Aged Cashew Cheese

★ Field Roast ~ Chao Slices

★ Follow Your Heart ~ Shredded, Sliced, Specialty & Blocks

★ Kite-Hill ~ Cream Cheese & Soft Spreadable Cheese Alternatives

★ Miyoko's Creamery ~ Farmhouse & Pepper Jack, Mozzarella, Cheese Wheels & Cream Cheese

★ Nona ~ Vegan Cheesy Sauces (Canada)

★ Parma ~ Vegan Parmesan

★ Parmela Creamery ~ Shreds & Slices

★ So Delicious ~ Dairy-Free Shreds

★ Treeline ~ Soft French-Style, Aged Artisanal & Cream Cheese

★ Violife ~ Blocks, Grated, Slices & Cream Cheese

★ Vromage ~ Various Artisan Styles

Internationally Distributed Dairy-Free Cheese Brands

* Europe, Canada, Brazil - Violife ~ Blocks, Grated, Slices & Cream Cheese
* UK - Applewood Vegan Cheese ~ Blocks & Slices
* UK - Tyne Chease Ltd ~ Various Artisan Styles
* UK - I Am Nut OK ~ Various Artisan Styles
* Scotland - Bute Island Sheese ~ Sheese Blocks, Slices, Grated & Cream Cheese Style

Eating Eggs Isn't What It's Cracked Up to Be

* The vast majority of egg-laying chickens are crammed into battery cages, where they have less room than a sheet of letter-size paper to live their entire lives from when they are hatched until when they are killed.

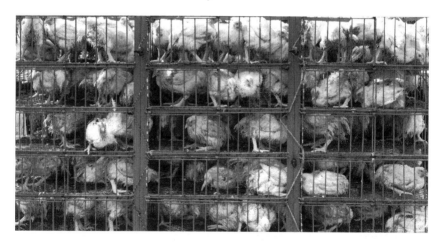

* These cages are made out of wire & stacked in such a way that the waste produced by the birds above falls through the wire floors onto the birds below. The stench is overpowering.

* Their beaks are cut off without anesthesia & they are also subjected to forced molting by shocking them through withholding food & water. Both of these routine practices are cruel & painful.

★ The baby male chicks are small & cannot lay eggs, so they are routinely ground up alive or slowly suffocated in dumpsters.

★ So, when you buy eggs from these factory egg farms, which is where 99% of eggs come from in the U.S, you are causing this suffering & ingesting this misery.

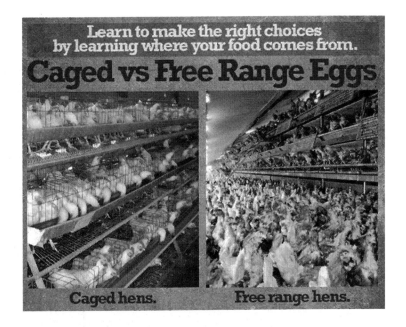

★ "Free range" in factory farms is not free! The term is legally undefined & tens of thousands of hens, though not in battery cages, are crammed into stinking warehouses with no fresh air or sunlight & forced to stand in their own excrement.

★ Less than 1% of chickens nationwide are raised as "free range," according to the National Chicken Council.

★ Ask yourself, would you like to be treated like this? Is any egg worth this?

* There are so many delicious & nutritious egg substitutes available today, such as: ground flax seeds, chia seeds, mashed bananas, apple sauce, silken tofu & Ener-G Egg Replacer.

* Remember, what goes around comes around, one way or another.

* Dairy & eggs are allergens, which cause symptoms such as asthma, respiratory problems, arthritis, clogging of the arteries & a host of other health issues.

* By eliminating dairy & eggs from your diet, you will feel better on all levels & contribute to the end of these insane & cruel ways of treating cows, goats & chickens.

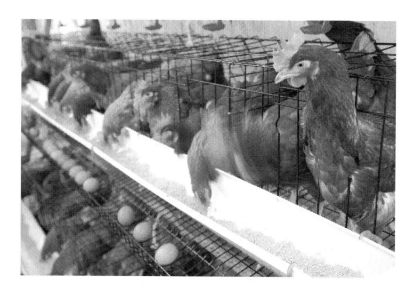

* Let's all remember & put into practice the Golden Rule. The Golden Rule is the principle of treating others as you want to be treated. It is a principle that is found in most religions & cultures worldwide. By implementing the Golden Rule, together, we can usher in a Golden Age.

Love Animals ~ Don't Eat Them!

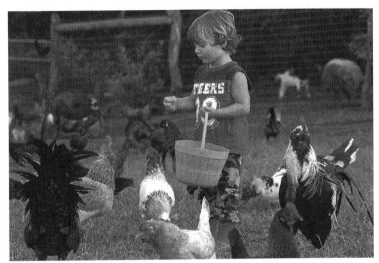

My precious friend Koa Le'amohala
at Leilani Farm Sanctuary, Maui, Hawaii.

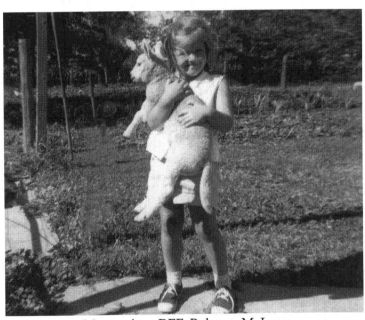

My precious BFF, Rebecca McLean,
loving a 'lambie' at age 5.

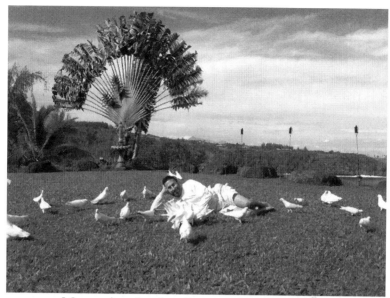
My precious brother, Swaroop Fredrick Honig,
the bird whisperer at TheGardens.org, Maui, Hawaii.

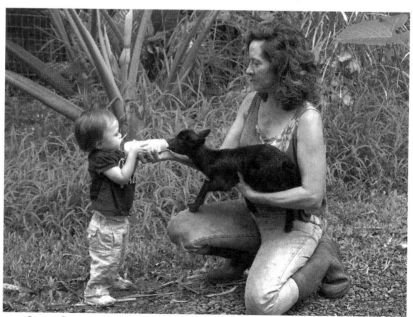
One of my precious vegan kindred Spirits, Laurelee Blanchard,
founder of Leilani Farm Sanctuary, Maui Hawaii.

"If you see yourself in others, then whom can you harm?"
- The Buddha

"Each time a person stands up for an ideal, or acts to improve the lot of others, they send forth a tiny ripple of hope... These ripples build a current which can sweep down the mightiest walls of oppression and resistance."
- Robert F. Kennedy

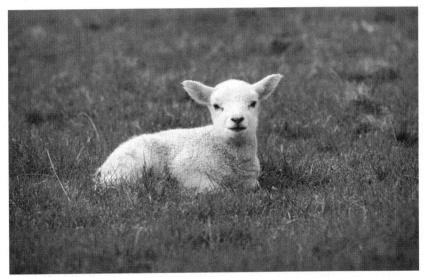

"I am not a cardigan or a chop. I am a living being, just like you."

"Animals are not ours to eat, wear, experiment on, or use for entertainment."
- PETA

"Until he extends his circle of compassion to include all living things, man will not himself find peace."
- Albert Schweitzer

"The magic moment is that in which a yes or no may change the whole of our existence."
- Paulo Coehlo

The Boomerang Effect

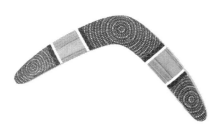

"The game of life is a game of boomerangs. Our thoughts, deeds & words return to us sooner or later with astounding accuracy."
- Florence Scovel Shinn

★ What goes around comes around.

★ We kill animals; we die of heart attacks.

★ We force-feed animals; we suffer with obesity.

★ We ingest the biochemistry of terror & misery from these abused animals; we suffer from anxiety & depression.

★ We rape animals through forced artificial insemination; women are raped worldwide.

★ We milk animals with painful electric machines; we suffer with breast cancer & contaminated breast milk.

★ We terrorize animals; we suffer from domestic violence & war.

★ We devastate our environment; GMOs, water shortages, pollution, fires & the climate crisis devastate us.

- ★ We rip away animals' babies hours after birth; our families are broken apart.

- ★ We enslave animals & modern-day slavery is running rampant.

- ★ We hyper confine animals in wet markets & in factory farms & now we find ourselves confined in lockdowns due to global pandemics.

- ★ We cut down forests, which are the lungs of our planet, for grazing cattle & growing crops to feed animals for meat & now our lungs are being attacked by respiratory diseases.

- ★ The good news is that all of this is reversible & we can avoid future strains of harmful viruses by going vegan! I elaborate on this in the upcoming segment about preventing future pandemics.

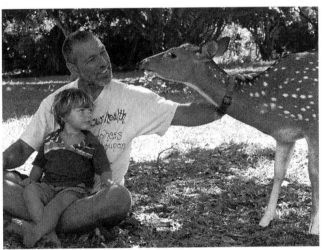

My precious friends, Home & Koa Le'amohala at Leilani Farm Sanctuary, Maui, Hawaii.

"I am not venison, I am Bambi."

The Bible states that "As you sow, so shall you reap." By replacing the mentality of domination & violence toward animals, with lovingkindness & cooperation, animal liberation becomes environmental liberation & human liberation.

It is high time to take off the blinders, connect the dots & ***go vegan!***

How to Prevent Future Pandemics

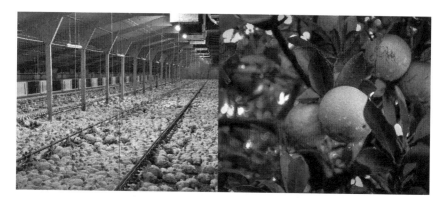

"Those who cannot remember the past are condemned to repeat it."
- George Santayana

As I have been saying for years & wrote in my last book, *Feel Good Now ~ How to Feel Your Best & Have Your Best to Give*, all of the major problems that we face on Earth today have their roots in cruelty to animals & can be reversed by going vegan!

Factory farms, slaughterhouses & wet markets, where animals are brutally confined, tortured & killed, are breeding grounds for infectious disease agents that create a storm environment for pandemics.

According to Dr. Michael Greger, humans have been on Earth for millions of years & yet throughout most of human evolution there were no epidemic diseases. People never got smallpox, measles, influenza, or even the common cold because those diseases did not even exist.

Medical anthropologists have identified three major periods of disease since the beginning of human evolution. The first began about 10,000 years ago with the domestication of animals.

Domestication may sound like a friendly word but what it actually means, in this context, is the imprisonment of animals. Animals were forcefully confined & abused for their meat, milk, skins & labor. Animals brought these diseases with them.

Confined, domesticated animals are breeding grounds for a wide range of diseases, many of which originally came from wild animals.

The 1918 Spanish Influenza, which was allegedly transferred from ducks to humans, reportedly infected 500 million people worldwide, which at that time was one third of the Earth's population. Reports indicate that more than 50 million people died of that disease with 675,000 in the United States.

The 1957 Asian Influenza that was reportedly transferred from birds to humans, caused an estimated one to two million deaths worldwide with 116,000 in the United States.

The 1968 Hong Kong Influenza, that was apparently transferred from poultry farms, reportedly killed one million people worldwide & around 100,000 people in the United States.

The 1981 HIV/AIDS that was allegedly transferred from chimpanzees has reportedly killed 38 million people worldwide.

In 2009, the deadly swine flu pandemic allegedly emerged from a massive pig farm in Veracruz, Mexico, where hundreds of pigs died from an outbreak that transferred to people. The CDC estimated that 51,700 - 575,400 people worldwide died from this H1N1 virus infection during the first year the virus circulated.

In August, 2010, the World Health Organization declared an end to the global 2009 H1N1 influenza pandemic. However, this virus continues to circulate as a seasonal flu virus & reportedly causes illness, hospitalization & deaths worldwide every year.

Medical historians state that we are currently in the third era of human infectious diseases & it is being called the age of emerging plagues. It includes diseases such as SARS, Ebola, HIV/AIDS, mad cow disease, E. coli, bird flu & other emerging diseases.

Humans kill live animals in wet meat markets & hyper-confine them in stockyards, factory farms & even in many smaller-scale operations, and now we have been confined in lockdowns & shelter-in-place conditions. Does anyone see the boomerang effect here?

Humans cut down trees that are the lungs of our planet to graze cattle & grow feed crops for them. According to many researchers, SARS-CoV-2 can trigger a respiratory tract infection. What goes around, comes around. As we sow, so shall we reap. This is also known as *karma*.

In poultry factory farms, tens of thousands of chickens are crammed into football stadium-sized sheds that are breeding grounds for disease. These birds are forced to stand in their own waste. The ammonia from the decomposition of their waste burns their lungs. (Is it any surprise that many diseases attack our lungs?) The stress from the sheer number of animals in these overcrowded conditions, combined with the lack of sunlight & fresh air, cripples the immune systems of these living beings.

Treating animals this way is tragic! If people don't have the conscience to shut down these concentration camps for animals, they will end up being shut down by an even deadlier pandemic.

Confining, torturing & killing animals, who have feelings like we do, is cruel.

Cruelty to cows ⟶ measles
Cruelty to camels ⟶ smallpox
Cruelty to pigs ⟶ whooping cough
Cruelty to water buffalo ⟶ leprosy
Cruelty to horses ⟶ the common cold
Cruelty to chickens ⟶ typhoid fever
Cruelty to ducks ⟶ the 1918 Spanish Influenza
Cruelty to chimpanzees ⟶ HIV-AIDS
Cruelty to birds & pigs ⟶ the swine flu
Cruelty to bats, civet cats, pangolins & other crammed animals ⟶ SARS

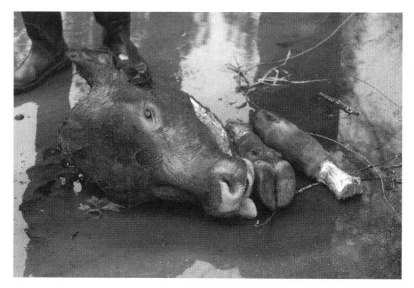

It is the consciousness of domination & violence that is the root cause of all of this suffering.

As Thoreau said, *"There are a thousand hacking at the branches of evil to one who is striking at the root."*

If the world had listened to vegan advocates, it is likely that coronaviruses & other zoonotic diseases since the domestication of animals could have been avoided. The good news is that future strains of harmful infectious diseases can be prevented.

In addition to preventing future pandemics, let's keep in mind that the underlying comorbidities, such as heart disease, type-2 diabetes, obesity, cancer & high blood pressure make us more susceptible to debilitating illness & death from these infectious diseases. By going vegan we can prevent, arrest & reverse these underlying conditions which gives us a better chance of surviving & thriving!

My beloved Gurudev, Sri Swami Satchidananda, said that karma is not a punishment; it is for our benefit & education.

Hopefully, the pandemics we have been experiencing will be an effective wake-up call for humanity. Prevention is better than cure. Disease, death & draconian health mandates may become commonplace in the world unless humans go vegan. The real "vaccine cure" is to stop abusing & consuming animals!

"Humanity needs to shift from being the tormentor to the mentor!"
- Meenakshi Angel Honig

Let's make this the year when humans wake up from this dark cultural trance & usher in a new era, from dis-ease to ease.

The good news is that there are soooo many delicious & nutritious plant-based options readily available, so it is easier than ever to transition to a plant-based diet!

The principle of *ahimsa* (non-violence) applies to every time period & to all situations. We are here to create history, not repeat it. By implementing *ahimsa* we can reverse so many problems. Therefore, for the sake of the animals, for human health, to prevent future pandemics & for survival of life on planet Earth ~ ***Let's Go Vegan!***

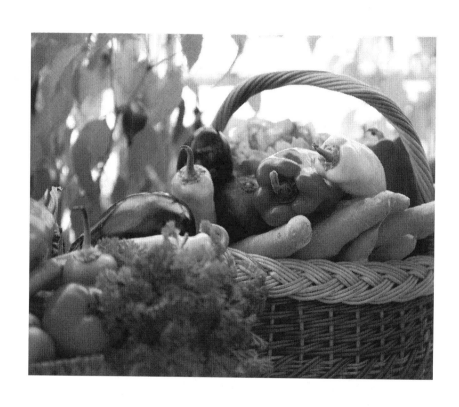

From Dissonance to Consonance
From Disconnection to Reconnection

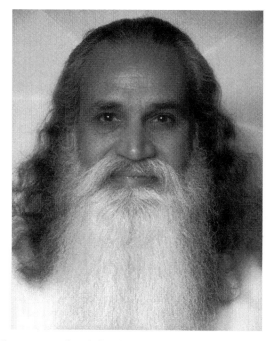

"The most cherished treasure in life is peace."
- Sri Swami Satchidananda

I had the astronomical blessing of meeting & studying with a world-renowned Yoga master, Sri Swami Satchidananda, from the age of 16.

I have been teaching Yoga & Meditation for nearly 50 consecutive years! One thing that I know for sure is that we are, by nature, peaceful.

That is why when anything disturbs our peace, we feel out of sorts with ourselves. We all naturally strive for harmony & balance.

Even our body temples are wired that way & are constantly striving for homeostasis, which refers to stability, balance & equilibrium within our cells.

Homeostasis is a dynamic equilibrium rather than a constant, unchanging state. It is a process involving continual monitoring of all systems in the body to detect changes & employing mechanisms that respond to those changes to restore stability.

Because we naturally strive for harmony & balance, both physically & psychologically, we find that when our attitudes & behaviors are not in alignment, a feeling of discomfort arises.

When our thoughts, attitudes, beliefs & values are not congruent with our actions, behaviors, habits & lifestyle, cognitive dissonance occurs.

This produces a feeling of discomfort that leads to an alteration in our attitudes, beliefs or behaviors to reduce the discomfort & to restore balance.

In an insightful article by Kendra Cherry, she points out that although cognitive dissonance can occur in many areas of life, it is particularly evident in situations where an individual's behavior conflicts with beliefs that are integral to their self-identity.

If you ask people if it morally correct to cause unnecessary suffering to animals, the vast majority of people will say no. And yet this same vast majority causes 72 billion land animals & over a trillion sea creatures to be tortured & killed for food each year.

How is this possible?

We strive for harmony and consistency with our values. So, in order to say that we love animals and are against animal cruelty, we have to disconnect in some way. This gives rise to the uncomfortable feeling of cognitive dissonance.

In an attempt to restore a feeling of peace & harmony, we use coping strategies such as rationalizing, justifying, trivializing, denying & euphemizing.

Here are some common euphemisms, just to name a few ~

★ Meat - instead of tortured, dead animals & rotting carcasses

★ Veal - instead of tortured baby cows

★ Pork, ham, bacon, sausage - instead of tortured, murdered pigs

★ Game - instead of hunted & killed wild animals

★ Beef & Steak - instead of tortured, murdered cows

★ Hot dogs - instead of ground up animal parts of cows, pigs & chickens, including skin, lips, pig snouts, organs, fat & other parts of animal bodies

★ Hamburger - instead of dead cows on a bun

★ Animal Agriculture & Factory Farms - instead of concentration & death camps for animals

★ Fowl - instead of foul play for birds

* Artificial insemination - instead of chained rape

* Harvesting - instead of murdering

* Broilers - instead of birds

* Cage-free - instead of cramped sheds & warehouses

* Free-range - instead of crammed sheds & warehouses with 1.2 square feet of floor space per hen

* Farrowing crates - instead of cages so small that the animals can't turn around or lie down comfortably in them

* Processing plants - instead of mass murder facilities

* Forced molting - instead of the cruel practice of starving hens in order to shock them into another laying cycle to increase output & profit

* Organic - instead of confined animals subjected to immense cruelty and painful deaths who cannot receive antibiotics to alleviate their suffering because the "organic" label yields a higher price

* Poultry service processor - instead of a torture device to debeak baby birds without anesthesia

* Depopulation methods - instead of gunshot, captive-bolt guns, electrocution & manual blunt-force trauma

* Fillers - instead of expired dog & cat food, poultry feces, blood, feathers & leftover restaurant food, among other things

★ Stanchions & feed racks - instead of structures to shackle and confine cows for forced impregnation and feeding so they will stay pregnant and produce babies and milk that are stolen from them

★ Humane - Seriously, is any of this humane???

Then we pack these abused, dead animals in foam trays with plastic wrap, physically, verbally & conceptually distancing ourselves from the real origin of this so-called food.

Just as hunger motivates us to find food to reduce our hunger, cognitive dissonance motivates us to find ways to reduce the dissonance. So, meat eaters can either stop eating meat or come up with reasons to justify why it is morally OK.

So, let's take a look at some of the common rationales that are encouraged in our culture to help us assuage the natural guilt we feel from being agents of horrific cruelty to animals, while claiming that we are animal lovers & how we might replace these rationalizations with a deeper truth.

Counter-questions Instead of Counter-attacks

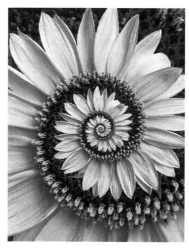

"The quality of your life is a direct reflection of the quality of the questions you are asking yourself."
- Tony Robbins

I was reflecting & contemplating upon the most common excuses that people give themselves for not going vegan, even when they are well aware of the horrors involved in the meat, dairy & egg industries. I was inspired to give a voice to these excuses with the hope that it would make this book more relatable, in that someone would read an excuse & say to themselves, "Oh, that's me!"

Then I respond to each of these common excuses to shed the light of awareness on them & provide a new perspective that will hopefully inspire a more compassionate & sustainable choice.

While in the process of doing research for this book, I came across a website entitled, *Discover Vegan* that was created by Imke and Georg. I was awe-struck by their brilliant approach of counter-questions instead of counter-attacks!

I absolutely love this approach because by asking pointed questions, people can come up with their own answers from within. Then they can own it more as their truth because it came from within them, rather than just hearing it from someone else.

So rather than reinvent the wheel, I contacted *Discover Vegan* and asked for their permission to quote them. Imke emailed me back & graciously gave her permission & blessings! I am so grateful to share their brilliant approach with you, which is interwoven with many modifications, adaptations & elaborations that I made.

Eating animal products is my personal choice.

★ What about the personal choice of an animal who wants to live? Have you considered his or her personal choice?

★ If someone makes the personal decision to mistreat a dog, is it morally acceptable because it was his or her personal choice?

★ Is it morally justifiable to rape someone because it is the rapist's personal choice?

★ Is it okay for a murderer to kill someone because it is his or her personal choice?

I love animals.

★ Do you really love animals when you pay someone to torture & kill them?

★ Would you say, "I love my children and I also pay someone to torture & murder them?"

* Do you have a pet? Would it be possible for you to love your dog & then kill & eat him or her?

I like the taste of meat.

* What taste is worth taking the life of a living being?

* Do you think that we need more than just palate pleasure to morally justify an act?

* Is it morally acceptable for someone to kill a dog if that person likes the taste?

* What is so special about human beings that our taste buds are more valuable than the life of an animal?

* Do you think you have to give up the taste of animal products by going vegan?

* Did you know that today there is a wide variety of vegan alternatives for meat, milk, cheese & eggs?

* Are you aware that as a vegan, you can still eat burgers, hot dogs, lasagna, cheese pizza, burritos, cake, cookies & ice cream that are made from plant sources?

* Did you know that as a vegan you can still experience all the tastes & textures that you are used to? The only difference is that they are made from plants; no dead body parts, no cholesterol, no hormones & no antibiotics.

* Are you aware that there are countless recipes for traditional foods that have been veganized & that many find them to taste even better, without all the misery & fear that is involved in the animal-sourced versions?

* So, is it possible that you won't be compromising taste, but rather you will be enjoying a higher taste that is in good taste on all levels?

It's necessary; I need the protein to stay healthy.

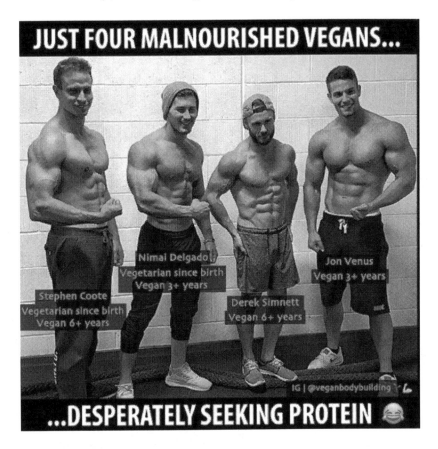

* Did you know that a peanut butter & jelly sandwich on whole grain bread contains 14 grams of protein whereas a McDonald's hamburger contains 13 grams of protein?

* Are you aware that research clearly shows that the SAD (Standard American Diet) causes an excess of protein?

* Did you know that our bodies take calcium from our bones in an attempt to neutralize this excess protein, contributing to such diseases as osteoporosis, arthritis & kidney failure, whereas a vegan diet provides all the protein that we need to be healthy & thrive without all the toxins & misery?

* Did you know that there is indisputable scientific evidence that consuming animal products has been inextricably linked to heart disease, type 2 diabetes, many forms of cancer, strokes, high blood pressure, dementia, osteoporosis & a host of other maladies?

* Are you aware that many of these diseases can be treated & even cured by switching to a plant-based diet?

* How can it be that both the American & the British Dietetic Association, the largest associations of nutrition experts in these countries, have declared that a vegan diet is suitable for all stages of life, including infancy, childhood, pregnancy, lactation, athletes & old-age?

* How can many athletes stay fit, strong & competitive if we need animal products to stay healthy?

* Here are some world class vegan athletes, just to name a few:

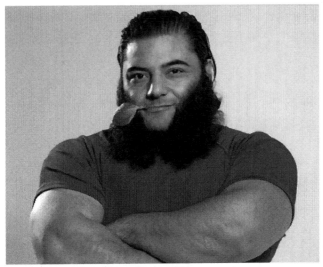

Patrik Baboumian ~ Vegan strongman

* Harri Nieminem ~ Boxer
* Pat Reeves ~ Powerlifter
* Alex Morgan ~ Soccer player
* Yolanda Presswood ~ Powerlifter
* Carl Lewis ~ Olympic sprinter
* Sofia Jokl ~ Ju-Jitsu expert
* Scott Jurek ~ Long-distance runner
* Lewis Hamilton ~ Formula 1 racing driver
* Venus Williams ~ Tennis player
* Jermain Defoe ~ Footballer
* David Haye ~ Boxer
* Barny du Plessis ~ Bodybuilder
* Hannah Teter ~ Snowboarder
* Kendrick Yahcob Farris ~ Weightlifter
* Tia Blanco ~ Surfer
* Nate Diaz ~ Mixed martial artist
* Jack Lindquist ~ Track cyclist
* Abel "Killa" Trujillo ~ Mixed martial artist
* Denis Mikhaylove ~ Ultradistance runner

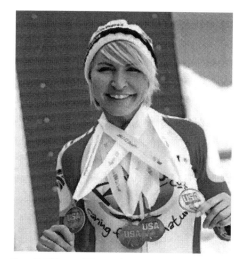

Heather Mills ~ Olympic 4 Gold-Medals Skier

* Borja Perez Batet ~ Runner
* Cody Elkins ~ Racquetball player
* Andy Lally ~ Racing driver
* Michaela Copenhaver ~ Rower
* Neil Robertson ~ Snooker player
* David Meyer ~ Martial artist
* Ruth Heidrich ~ Endurance athlete
* Alexander Dargatz ~ Bodybuilder
* Fiona Oakes ~ Marathon runner

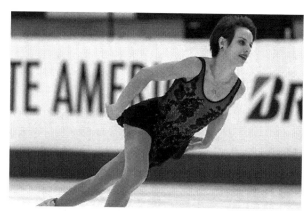

Meagan Duhamel ~ Olympic Gold-Metal Figure Skater

I can't live without cheese.

★ Did you know that dairy cheese is made from milk that causes gruesome pain to dairy cows, rips away their babies at birth, causes greenhouse gasses that significantly contribute to climate destabilization and pollute the air, soil & water supply?

★ Are you aware that even though dairy is advertised to be this pure white substance, it is actually filled with blood, pus, antibiotics, toxins, misery, cholesterol & fat, all of which contribute to asthma, allergies, respiratory problems, heart disease, cancer & a host of other ailments?

★ Did you know that even though dairy is purported to be good for your bones, it actually leaches calcium from your bones & contributes to osteoporosis?

★ Given that there are so many non-dairy cheeses readily available today that taste even better without all the toxins, misery & detrimental effects on our health, do you think a better question would be, *"How can I live **with** dairy cheese?"*

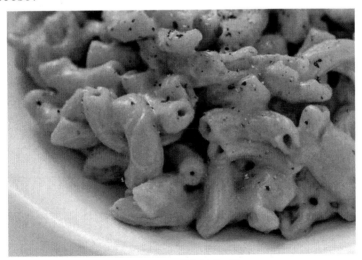

Creamy Vegan Mac & Cheese

Eating meat is part of our tradition & culture.

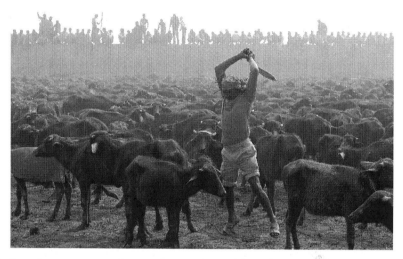

* Just because we have done something for many years or even centuries, does that justify its existence & continuation?

* Slavery, racial segregation, the oppression of women & gay people were once regarded as a tradition & part of our culture. Is that a valid reason for continuing practices of oppression?

* Bullfights are considered to be a strong part of the tradition in Spain, as is the slaughter of dolphins in Taiji, the dog meat festival in Yulin & the world's largest animal sacrifice, the Gadhimai festival in Nepal. Does this mean that these cruel, gut-wrenching practices should continue to exist because they are part of a culture or tradition?

* Did you know that cannibalism is very much still alive today despite being considered repulsive by the vast majority of societies? There are areas where eating human flesh is ingrained in tradition and is part of the culture. Would it be OK to torture, kill & eat *you* because this is a part of a traditional cultural ritual?

Our ancestors ate meat.

★ Do you think that history is justification? Do you think that just because our ancestors did something, that makes it right? Our ancestors did a lot of things that we don't do today.

★ If it is morally acceptable to eat animals because our ancestors did it, does that mean that it is morally acceptable to kill each other because our ancestors did?

★ Do you think our actions should be evaluated on their merit & demerit or merely based on the fact that it was done in the past?

Some wild animals eat meat.

★ So, are you a wild animal?

★ Wild animals kill each other. Does that mean it's morally acceptable for people to kill each other?

★ Animals kill their own food; they don't pay someone else to do it for them. Do you?

★ Did you know that according to a new survey by Cherry Digital, an international PR company, nearly half of the meat eaters in the United States would rather go vegetarian than kill an animal themselves for food? The survey data revealed that 49.3 % of the population would not eat meat if they personally had to take the life of an animal.

★ Carnivores such as lions & tigers need to eat meat to survive. Do you need to eat meat to survive? If not, why do you do it?

★ Humans have a moral compass. Do you think it is up to us to make ethical choices?

★ Given that our benevolent Creator has graciously given us every nutrient that we need to thrive from the plant kingdom, why would a compassionate person harm animals unnecessarily?

If we stop eating animals, wouldn't they take over the planet or die out?

★ Are you aware that the only reason we have so many animals is because we breed billions of animals every year on a massive scale through artificial insemination for meat, dairy & eggs? Do you think that if we stop breeding them, the Earth would return to its natural balance of human animals & non-human animals?

★ Animal husbandry is based on supply & demand. When we demand it, they supply it. Farmers only breed as many animals as they can sell. So, what are they going to do when we stop buying them?

★ Did you know that industrial animal husbandry is the main cause of the greatest mass extinction in the last 65 million years?

★ If you are concerned about preventing species extinction, wouldn't it be a good idea to go vegan & inspire others to do the same?

I like the way that eating meat makes me feel.

★ Did you know that when we are not filling our body temples with the biochemistry of misery & terror that comes from ingesting tortured & murdered living beings, and when we are not disturbing our peace with the cognitive dissonance that results from not living in alignment with our true values of kindness, we feel much better?

★ Are you aware that one out of six Americans is taking anti-depressant drugs? Do you think there is any connection between people ingesting the misery of tortured animals & feeling miserable?

★ Did you know that eating meat is one of the major causes of heart disease, cancer, diabetes & a host of other diseases? Does having those diseases make you feel good?

★ Does caring for & losing loved ones with those diseases make you feel good?

★ Did you know that a vegan diet is the healthiest diet for your mind, body, spirit & for planet Earth?

★ Did you know that, *"Nothing tastes as good as vegan feels!"*?

Human rights are more important than animal rights.

★ Did you know that 82% of starving children live in countries where food is grown to feed livestock in richer countries?

★ Are you aware that becoming vegan would put an end to this unjust distribution of food?

★ Why is it that we have enough food to feed 72 billion land animals every year & yet according to the United Nations Food & Agriculture Organization, 815 million people are suffering from chronic malnourishment?

★ Why does the fact that there are homeless people or starving children make it acceptable for you to pay someone to torture & slaughter animals?

Animals don't feel pain & suffer the way that we do.

★ Did you know that both land animals & sea animals have nervous systems & are therefore able to feel physical pain?

★ Have you ever stepped on the tail of a dog? Do you think the dog was in pain or not?

★ Are you aware that it has been documented that animals experience emotional suffering, just like humans do?

★ Do you think that mother cows mourn the loss of their kidnapped calves, that orcas grieve for their abducted offspring & dogs suffer from separation anxiety when their human companions leave them alone?

That's the food chain.

★ In nature, food chains exist because predators must kill their prey in order to survive. Do you have to kill someone to survive?

★ We breed animals selectively, artificially inseminate them, drag them into trucks, dismember them & slaughter them. Is that what you think a natural food chain looks like?

★ So, are you saying that *"might makes right?"* In your code of ethics, is it morally acceptable for us to enslave & exploit others because we have the physical ability to do so?

★ Do you think it is right for people to inflict acts of cruelty based on the illusion of self-assigned superiority? Is it right that one religion is believed to be superior to another religion, or one race is believed to be superior to another race, or human animals are believed to be superior to non-human animals?

★ Is a false sense of self-proclaimed superiority justification for causing harm to others?

We're smarter than animals.

★ Does intelligence define the value of a life?

★ Is your life worth more than that of a mentally challenged person or a child whose intellect is not as developed as yours?

★ If intelligence means dominance, does that mean that any person with a high IQ can do whatever they want to a person with a lower IQ?

★ There are different types of intelligence, so who decides that "IQ" is the gold standard for measuring intelligence anyway?

★ A pig has the same cognitive abilities & intelligence as a three-year-old child. Does this mean that from now on you will eat toddlers instead of pigs?

Without us, animals would not live at all, so they should be grateful to us.

★ Do you think you could go into a slaughterhouse, look an animal in the eye right before he or she is being killed & tell that animal to thank you for his or her life?

★ If I breed a dog & then abuse & kill him, am I a good person because this dog would not have been born had I not bred him?

★ If a child is born into a violent family where he or she is confined, abused & eventually killed would you think, "Well, at least the child's parents gave him or her the chance to live?"

Can't we just improve the lives of animals?

★ Do you think the animals who are kept on small farms are petted to death?

★ Did you know that undercover footage of small backyard operations typically reveals horrific abuse of animals?

★ What happens to the babies of these animals & what happens to dairy cows when their milk production declines?

★ Do you think that dogs should be treated better in dog meat factories in China & killed in a more "humane" way?

★ Would a golden retriever steak with an animal welfare label be acceptable to you?

We stun the animals before we kill them so they don't feel a thing.

* Did you know that animals are dragged into slaughterhouses where they are terrorized by what they see, feel & smell?

* Did you know that due to the pressure to process animals quickly, many animals fail to be anesthetized properly & are fully conscious when they are killed & cut open?

* Can we kill an animal in a humane way? Aren't killing & humane contradictory terms?

* Jeffrey Dahmer was a serial killer who drugged his victims before he killed them. Does this mean that he was a good person who cared for the welfare & humane treatment of his victims?

Animals are bred for this purpose.

* Does this mean that dog fights are moral because these animals were bred for this purpose?

* In Africa, lions are bred so that big-game hunters can shoot them. Is the hunter therefore acting morally because the animal was bred for that purpose?

Plants have feelings, too.

* Yes, plants do have feelings, but do plants have the same brain and central nervous system that animals have?

★ In the name of *ahimsa*, (non-violence) should we do our best to cause the minimal amount of pain possible to the creatures with whom we co-habitat this beautiful Earth?

★ If a dog jumps in front of your car, would you dodge into a lawn or run over the dog?

★ It takes up to 16 pounds of grain to make one pound of meat. So, if you care that much about plants, why not skip the inefficient process of cycling the grains through the animal & eat them directly?

★ Are you aware that eating plant food is both more efficient & more compassionate to all?

I can't be 100% Vegan.

★ Imagine if the coastguard sees a group of children drowning but it is not possible to save all of them in time. Should they just turn around & let everyone drown because they can't save 100%? Or should they at least try to save some children?

What if you were stranded on a desert island?

★ Due to the exploding number of vegans stranded on desert islands, there will soon be vegan supermarkets on all desert islands! :)

★ Wouldn't this be a better question to ask: If you are living in a location where there is plenty of food & you just have to go to any supermarket or health food store to find an abundance of delicious, healthy vegan food, why would you choose food that causes massive deforestation, global warming, habitat loss, species extinction, pollution, unnecessary violent deaths of innocent animals, starving children & a decline in your own health, given that it is completely unnecessary?

I am in the habit of eating meat.

★ Are you aware that our thoughts affect our words, our words affect our actions, our actions affect our habits, our habits affect our character & our character affects our destiny?

★ Do you think that changing your habit of eating meat will affect your character & destiny?

★ Did you know that first you form your habits & then your habits form you?

★ Do you think it better to choose habits that result in cruelty, disease & destruction or habits that result in lovingkindness, health & sustainability?

★ Are you in charge of your habits? Can you decide to change your habits if you become aware of better ones?

It takes too much time.

★ Are you aware that there are countless vegan recipes that are readily available that take less than 30 minutes to prepare?

* Did you know that there are a multitude of videos on YouTube that demonstrate how to prepare quick, delicious & nutritious vegan meals?

* Are you aware that you can prepare quick vegan meals in an instant pot, air fryer, crock pot, toaster oven, rice cooker, blender & Vitamix?

* Did you know that eating raw vegan food can be quick, easy, nutritious & super yum? Have you ever seen Fully Raw Kristina's YouTube channel?

* Did you know that you can even get vegan fast food? (Not that I recommend it.) Here are some options, just to name a few ~

    * Burger King Impossible Whopper & French toast Sticks
    * McDonalds has 7 vegan options
    * Subway Beyond Meatball Marinara
    * Carl's Jr. French Fries
    * Domino's Thin Crust Pizza
    * Taco Bell Black Bean Crunchwrap Supreme
    * Hardee's Beyond Breakfast Sausage Biscuit
    * Wendy's Plain Baked Potato
    * Papa John's Breadsticks
    * Panera Baja Grain Bowl
    * Panda Express Chow Mein & Eggplant tofu
    * Auntie Anne's Sweet Almond Pretzel
    * Baskin-Robbins Nondairy Ice Cream
    * Starbucks offers several vegan options
    * Chipotle is great for all kinds of dietary restrictions because you can mix & match all the ingredients yourself.

★ Did you know that on PETA's website there is an entire directory of fast food options?

★ Are you aware that there are phone apps to help you find quick vegan food near you, such as *Happy Cow*? (This makes it super easy when you are traveling!)

★ Did you know that there is a resource section at the end of this book for further info?

Morality is subjective.

★ Then ask yourself, "Would I want that inflicted on me? If not, what right do I have to do it to others?"

★ If morality is subjective, what sense does our legal system have? Any behavior would be acceptable, wouldn't it?

★ Would it be acceptable if I beat & kill a cat because I think it is morally correct?

My mother thinks that my kids will be weak & brain dead if they don't eat meat.

★ Are you aware that it has been scientifically shown that a vegan diet is healthier for people of all ages?

★ Did you know that the Physicians Committee for Responsible Medicine has an illuminating section on its website that offers a wealth of information on plant-based diets specifically for infants, children & teens?

★ Are you aware that PETA offers a comprehensive guide for vegan nutrition for kids?

★ Did you know that kids are happier & healthier when they live in alignment with *ahimsa* (non-violence) & have reverence for all life?

Isn't it enough to be a vegetarian?

★ What do you think happens to the male calves in the dairy industry?

★ What happens to male chicks in egg production given that they don't give eggs & they're not suitable for meat production?

★ Don't you think it's strange that humans are the only species that drinks milk from another species?

★ Do you think it is strange that humans are the only adults who drink milk after being weaned as a child?

★ Do you think that rat milk is for baby rats, kangaroo milk is for baby kangaroos, dog milk is for baby dogs but that cow milk & goat milk is for baby & adult humans??

★ Would you suck on a cow's udder or on the mammary gland of a rat?

★ Do you think it is OK for dairy cows to be raped & have their babies stolen from them at birth so that you can drink their milk that was intended for their calves?

★ How would you feel if your babies were stolen from you at birth after carrying them for 9 months, just like a mother cow does?

* Would you like to be forced to endure having painful metal machines on your breasts to steal your milk that was intended for your baby that had just been ripped away from you?

* Would you want to be treated that way?

* Do realize that what goes around comes around?

* Do realize that you have a choice?

* Did you know that there are countless non-dairy substitutes readily available that are delicious & nutritious without this pain & misery?

* What do you think is the right choice?

Some Yoga teachers eat dairy & some Yoga ashrams serve dairy products.

* If a Yoga teacher drinks alcohol & smokes cigarettes, would that make it a healthy choice for you to do the same?

* If you are a Yoga teacher who teaches *ahimsa*, (non-violence) do you think that your dietary choices should be congruent with your teachings?

* Or, is it OK to teach *ahimsa* & then buy, serve & ingest dairy products that directly cause horrific violence, which is the opposite of *ahimsa*?

* What rationalizations do you give yourself to justify that?

* Are those rationalizations based on *satya* (truthfulness)?

★ Is consuming dairy products in alignment with *asteya* (non-stealing)?

★ Do you think it is better to blindly follow "tradition" or to put on your critical thinking cap & make dietary choices that are congruent with *ahimsa*, (non-violence), *satya*, (truthfulness) & *asteya*, (non-strealing)?

★ Do you think that Yoga is an evolving science?

★ Is it better to perpetuate traditions that cause suffering or to evolve those traditions in ways that are in alignment with the foundational practice of *ahimsa*, which is the first *yama* or ethical principle, upon which the entire science of Yoga rests?

Farmers & livestock producers would lose their jobs.

★ Do you think their jobs are more important than the lives of animals & the future of our planet?

★ Would you encourage someone to smoke cigarettes just because the tobacco farmers & the people who work in the cigarette industry could lose their jobs?

★ Why do you think the jobs of livestock farmers are more important than those of tobacco farmers?

★ You're right, we must consider the livelihoods of people involved in animal agriculture. They are often born into agriculture, know no other way of life & have never questioned the morality of what they are doing. The farmers & livestock producers are doing a job that's being asked of them. They fulfill the wishes of consumers. How do our choices affect this?

* Do you think that the efforts that someone involved in animal agriculture has to make to find a new job is worse than enduring a life of suffering & fear that is inflicted on billions of animals?

* Are you concerned about the jobs of the slaughterhouse workers, too?

* Did you know that slaughterhouse workers, people who kill living beings for a living, kill hundreds or thousands of animals in a day?

* Did you know this repetitive stress causes a variety of disorders such as PTSD (post-traumatic stress disorder) & PITS (perpetration-induced traumatic stress)?

* Are you aware that when people suffer from these disorders it leads to an increase in crime rates, including higher incidents of domestic abuse, as well as alcohol & drug abuse?

* Do you think that your dietary choices & voting dollars, that are based on supply & demand, have anything to do with this?

* How about if they grow avocados & oranges instead?

It's too limiting to be a vegan.

* Do you think that it is limiting to billions of animals to be confined from when they are born until they are slaughtered?

★ Did you know that many people who switch to a vegan diet discover a wide variety of foods & spices that they never even knew existed?

★ Did you know that as a vegan, you can still eat pizza, spaghetti, burgers, fries, milkshakes, ice cream & cheese? The only difference is they are sourced from plants rather than tortured animals.

★ Have you considered that the vegan version is also free of the pesticides, antibiotics, toxins & the biochemistry of terror that is contained in the animal sourced version of these products?

Being vegan is extreme.

★ Do you think it is more extreme to eat tortured, murdered animals & their secretions than it is to eat fruit, vegetables, grains, legumes, nuts & seeds?

★ Isn't it more extreme to eat dead corpses that are sometimes weeks old?

★ Do you think it is more extreme to eat plant-based foods, or to have double, triple or quadruple coronary bypass surgery?

★ Do you think it's extreme to kill someone just because you like the taste of their legs or breasts?

★ How can a vegan diet be extreme if it consists of eating foods that prevent & cure diseases?

★ Do you think it is extreme to be an agent of horrific cruelty to countless animals & to contribute to starvation, environmental devastation, rainforest destruction, soil depletion & pollution by eating meat, eggs & dairy when there are many delicious & nutritious plant-based alternatives?

★ Do you think it is extreme to care more about a hamburger than the prevention of future pandemics & the survival of our planet, given that the climate crisis can be reversed by vegan dietary choices?

I only eat a little bit of meat.

★ That's great that you've reduced your consumption of animal products. What inspired you to reduce your meat consumption?

★ Have you ever thought that you still are paying for animals to be exploited & slaughtered – even if you consume less than before?

★ This is a good step in the right direction, but do you think that the animal who died for your Sunday roast is grateful to you for eating less meat?

★ That animal was killed & his or her life is over. Does your reduction change that fact?

I only eat meat on special occasions.

★ What makes an occasion special? Is that a free pass to cause suffering to others?

★ If something is a special occasion, wouldn't a better way of celebrating it be to be an instrument of lovingkindness & sustainability, rather than an agent of cruelty & devastation?

★ Wouldn't expressing your compassion for all life make the occasion even more special?

Being vegan is too expensive.

★ Have you noticed that when you go to a supermarket, the most expensive foods tend to be meat & cheese, whereas the less expensive foods such as grains, beans, potatoes, pasta, vegetables & fruits are vegan?

★ While it may be true that vegan meat substitutes can be expensive, could it be due to the fact they are often from smaller, mainly organic producers.

★ Did you know that the American government spends $38 billion each year to subsidize the meat & dairy industries, but only 0.04% of that ($17 million) each year to subsidize fruits & vegetables?

★ Do you think that when more people go vegan & buy more vegan products, they will become less expensive?

★ Did you know that your risk of heart disease & cancer, the two leading causes of death, are significantly reduced by a vegan diet?

★ Have you considered how much your poor health, missed time at work & hospitalizations will cost you due to consuming animal products?

* Did you know that the Dean Ornish Program, which is based on a low-fat vegan diet, reverses heart disease & cancer?

* Have you considered the cost of not being able to be with your loved ones and to do what you love because you are out of commission with diseases that can be reversed by a vegan diet?

Why do vegans eat stuff that looks like meat?

* Do you season, marinate & cook your meat? Why shouldn't vegans do the same with tofu, seitan, tempeh, jackfruit, taro, mushrooms, etc.?

* Many people did not go vegan because they no longer liked the taste of animal products. So why should they give up the taste, if no animals have to suffer for it?

* Why does the meat industry package meat in the form of a cucumber & call it sausage?

God made animals for us to eat.

* Do slaughterhouses look like the work of God or the work of the devil?

* If we don't have to kill God's creatures to survive, don't you think a kind, compassionate God would prefer that we not kill them?

* Isn't one of the 10 Commandments, *"Thou shall not kill"*?

* What is our right relationship with the Earth & with animals? Is it to be nature guardians? Are we here to protect & nurture or to torture & destroy?

* What kind of God would want you to enslave, rape & murder billions of innocent animals who feel pain just as you do when it is totally unnecessary?

* Do all spiritual paths teach the Golden rule which means, *"Do unto others as you would have them do unto you"*?

* 99% of meat, dairy & eggs comes from factory farms where animals are routinely confined, dehorned, debeaked, castrated & tortured from the moment that they are born until they are dragged off to a slaughter house. Is that the way you would like to be treated?

* If not, why pay other people to treat animals that way by consuming meat, dairy & eggs?

* Using a religious belief to justify killing animals is the same as using this belief to oppress woman, gay people & minorities.

Eating meat is our nature.

* Would you kill an animal yourself or would you find that repulsive or traumatizing? If it were our nature to eat meat, we would have no problem killing an animal.

* Have you ever seen an animal that was hit by a car? Did the sight of his torn organs make your mouth water? No? A real meat-eater would gobble it at once.

* Imagine being locked in a room with a live chicken & an apple. What would you eat first?

* When you see a "prey" animal, do you feel hungry? Do you have this instinct?

★ If it were natural to eat meat, wouldn't we teach our children to kill when they are young, like predators do with their young?

It's natural ~ people have always eaten meat. Why stop now?

★ Do you think that it is natural to evolve?

★ Given that 99% of meat dairy & eggs come from factory farms that cause horrific cruelty to animals, devastate the environment & cause both physical & psychological diseases to humanity, do you think it would be natural to rethink this & consider making more compassionate & sustainable choices?

★ Do you think that the nature of evolution is that when we know better we do better?

★ Have you ever considered this quote by Thomas Edison? *"Non-violence leads to the highest ethics, which is the goal of all evolution. Until we stop harming all other living beings, we are still savages."*

★ Would you rather be a force for ethical evolution or be a savage?

It's normal. Almost everyone eats meat & I don't want to be different.

★ What do you think Krishnamurti meant when he said, *"It is no measure of health to be well adjusted to a profoundly sick society."*?

★ How do you feel when you read this quote by Dr. Martin Luther King, Jr.? *"On some positions cowardice asks the question, is it safe? Expediency asks the question, is it politic? Vanity asks the question, is it popular? But conscience asks the question, is it right? There comes a time when one must take a position that is neither safe, nor politic, nor popular but he must take it because conscience tells him it is right."*

★ Do you think that normalizing a behavior makes it right?

★ Would you rather be normal or create a new normal that is based on health, sustainability & lovingkindness toward all?

I want a sense of belonging.

★ Do you think it is important to have a sense of belonging to your own true nature, which is kind & compassionate?

★ Did you know that the vegan movement is one of the fastest growing movements in the world today?

★ Are you aware that you can experience a sense of belonging by joining or starting vegan meet-up groups in your area?

★ Did you know that there are countless online vegan groups that you can join such as, Dr. Will Tuttle's *World Peace Diet Circle*, vegan groups on Facebook, vegan dating sites & so forth?

★ Are you aware that you can experience a sense of belonging by hosting or joining vegan potlucks, vegan book clubs & vegan movie nights?

★ Did you know that you can experience a sense of belonging by investing in plant-based substitutes for animal-based products & that this is one of the fastest-growing business opportunities?

★ Did you know that you can experience a sense of belonging by visiting an animal farm sanctuary & volunteering for local animal charities?

★ How about locating the closest vegetarian/vegan society near you & forming new friendships with people who genuinely care about animals, the environment & human health?

★ How about contacting me? I offer online coaching & personalized vegan retreats! :):)

Blood Type

★ There is a myth going around that people should base their diets on their blood types. Is it true that blood type O is traced back to cavemen, who were meat eaters, so type O individuals should eat meat?

★ Do you think that being an agent of horrific cruelty & ingesting the biochemistry of trauma & misery is beneficial for *any* blood type?

★ Is it a surprise that one in six Americans take some kind of psychiatric drugs — mostly antidepressants?

★ Do you think there is a cause & effect relationship between causing & ingesting misery & feeling miserable?

★ Did you know that a systemic scientific review of the evidence used to support the blood type diet denies its validity?

I like to make the same lasagna recipe that my grandmother made. It is comfort food for me.

★ Many traditional recipes for lasagna contain ground beef, pork sausage & dairy products. Is your "comfort" more important than the agonizing pain & suffering of cows & pigs?

★ Does causing & ingesting the biochemistry of terror & misery bring you true comfort? Do you understand that what goes around, comes around?

★ If I said that my traditional recipe for lasagna contained a quarter pound of golden retriever, would that be comfort food for you?

★ Do cows, pigs & golden retrievers all have the same central nervous systems & ability to feel pain?

* Do you think carrying on the tradition of our grandparents' recipes is justification for inflicting blood-curdling atrocities onto precious innocent animals?

* Did you know that you can veganize any traditional recipe from virtually all international cuisines in ways that are delicious, nutritious & kind?

* Would you rather be traditional or kind & on the right side of history?

Our canine teeth show that we were made to eat meat.

* Have you seen the research that humans are naturally plant-based eaters? Our physiology evolved for processing starches, fruits & vegetables, not tearing & chewing flesh.

* Did you know that a carnivore's teeth are long, sharp, pointed & designed to pierce flesh?

* Are you aware that humans, as well as other herbivore's teeth, are not pointed, but flat edged which are designed for biting, crushing & grinding?

* Have you ever read this essay by Plutarch? *"A human body in no way resembles those that were born for ravenousness; it hath no hawk's bill, no sharp talon, no roughness of teeth, no such strength of stomach or heat of digestion, as can be sufficient to convert or alter such heavy and fleshy fare. But if you will contend that you were born to an inclination to such food as you have now a mind to eat, do you then yourself kill what you would eat. But do it yourself, without the help of a chopping-knife, mallet or axe, as wolves, bears, and lions do, who*

kill and eat at once. Rend an ox with thy teeth, worry a hog with thy mouth, tear a lamb or a hare in pieces, and fall on & eat it alive as they do. But if thou had rather stay until what thou eat is to become dead, and if thou art loath to force a soul out of its body, why then dost thou against nature eat an animate thing? There is nobody that is willing to eat even a lifeless and a dead thing even as it is; so they boil it, and roast it, and alter it by fire and medicines, as it were, changing & quenching the slaughtered gore with thousands of sweet sauces, that the palate being thereby deceived may admit of such uncouth fare."

★ Do you still think that you were made to eat meat?

One person alone can't make a difference.

★ Are you going to vote? Why do you do that when one person can't make a difference?

★ Are you aware of the principle of supply & demand? Every time we buy vegan products, we change the demand & vote for the kind of world in which we'd like to live.

★ What would have happened if Mahatma Gandhi, Nelson Mandela, Rosa Parks or Dr. Martin Luther King, Jr. had said something like that? Sometimes it only takes one person to make a difference & inspire thousands or millions.

* If everyone had the attitude that one person cannot make a difference, then we would still have slavery, apartheid, woman would not be allowed to vote, same sex marriages would be prohibited, etc. It was precisely because individuals, who represented a minority at that time, got involved & spoke out against injustices, that change was brought about. Isn't it now up to us to do exactly the same to save the animals, the planet, ourselves & pave the way for future generations?

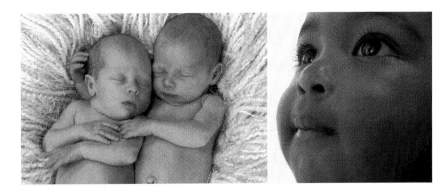

I don't know how to go vegan.

* Do think that where there is a will there is a way?

* Did you know that there are tons of great resources readily available about how to go vegan?

* Are you aware that at the end of this book there is a resource section to provide you with some valuable resources to get started!

* Did you know that you can arrange a coaching call with me & I can help you to tailor a graceful transition that is in harmony with your unique lifestyle? www.AngelYoga.com

"You have just dined & however scrupulously the slaughterhouse is concealed in the graceful distance of miles, there is complicity."
- Ralph Waldo Emerson

"Silence is consent." - Plato

Do you realize that we all have been brainwashed? As Dr. Julia Shaw said, *"Hypocrisy flourishes in social & cultural environments. Social habits can cast a veil over our moral conflicts, by normalizing our behavior."*

It is high time to re-think how we treat human beings, animals & the planet & acknowledge our own hypocrisies. Rather than doing mental gymnastics to justify unethical behavior, how about just making new choices?

"Veganism is not about giving anything up or losing anything; it is about gaining the peace within yourself that comes from embracing nonviolence & refusing to participate in the exploitation of the vulnerable."
- Gary L. Francione

By identifying & addressing even just a few of these ethical inconsistencies, we become healthier & happier people & the planet becomes a safer & kinder place to be! Would you rather be part of the problem or part of *the Soulution*?

My Wish to Protect Fish!

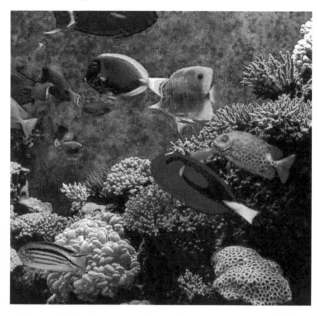

"Let's not be remiss in transforming an ocean of devastation into an ocean of bliss!"
- Meenakshi Angel Honig

Recently, I have spoken to several people who have told me that they are mostly vegan but they do eat fish, at times. It is particularly gut wrenching when I hear this from the mouths of Yoga teachers.

As I mentioned earlier, I have been teaching Yoga for nearly 50 consecutive years & by the time you read this, it may be over a half of a century! I am also a Yoga Teacher Trainer, meaning that I certify other people to become Yoga teachers.

Many people who call themselves Yoga teachers are actually *asana* teachers, meaning that they teach the physical postures but may have little or no understanding of the entire science of Yoga. Yoga is rooted in the foundation of ethical perfection as outlined in the *Yamas* & *Niyamas* in the *Yoga Sutras*.

The *Yamas & Niyamas* are 10 guidelines for ethical perfection upon which the entire science of Yoga is based. The first & foremost of these 10 guidelines is *Ahimsa* (nonviolence).

Additionally, given that I live on Maui where scuba diving, snorkeling and swimming with dolphins & whales is a highlight, it is painful to witness the cognitive dissonance of people raving about their experiences with these amazing sea creatures & then going out to lunch for fish tacos & out to dinner to seafood restaurants.

So, I feel compelled to shine the light of awareness on this vitally important topic. Eating fish is an unnecessary violation of *ahimsa* (non-violence). It causes massive animal suffering, ocean devastation & has a negative impact on our physical & moral health.

Let's take a look at these 3 areas. I would like to thank & acknowledge PETA, *Vegan.com* & Dr. Michael Klaper for elucidating many of these key points.

Animal Cruelty

Are fish animals?

★ The five most well-known classes of vertebrates (animals with backbones) are mammals, birds, fish, reptiles & amphibians.

★ A fish is an animal who lives & breathes in water.

★ There is clear evidence that fish feel pain & show fear.

★ Neurobiologists have long recognized that fish have nervous systems that comprehend & respond to pain.

* Fish, like other vertebrates, have neurotransmitters such as endorphins that relieve suffering. The only reason for their nervous systems to produce these painkillers is to alleviate pain.

* The science is clear that fish exhibit thinking skills & empathy.

* A 2017 study published in *Nature* indicates that fish rely on social interaction & community to deal with stressful occurrences.

* Almost every commercially-caught fish dies from suffocation.

* When fish are caught in deep waters & pulled to the surface, this depressurization can cause their organs to burst or their stomachs to protrude from their mouths.

* According to Dr. Michael Klaper, "Fish have highly developed nervous systems & feel severe pain from handling as well as suffocation when taken out of the water. The ethical equivalent of "sport fishing" has been described as hooking a dog in the jaw with a hamburger-baited hook & then dragging him or her underwater until he or she drowns. The exciting tugs of the fishline that so thrills the sportsman are the anguished efforts of a terrified animal struggling for his or her life."

* Whenever you purchase fish & seafood you are paying someone to torture animals which causes massive animal suffering.

* There are countless plant-based products, readily available today, that capture the tastes & textures of fish. This makes it sooo easy & delicious to switch to a more compassionate & sustainable choice!

Bycatch

★ Bycatch refers to the unwanted animals who are netted or hooked, then typically thrown back into the water dead.

★ Bycatch is all-pervasive in the fishing industry & its victims include fish, sea turtles, sea-birds, porpoises, dolphins, whales, etc.

★ If you've heard of the term *"dolphin-safe tuna"* it's because dolphins are frequently suffocated in nets laid by shrimp boats.

★ In the shrimp industry, there can be up to 20 pounds of bycatch for each pound of harvested shrimp!

★ When you purchase fish, you are causing massive suffering & death to countless other sea creatures, in addition to the fish that you are consuming.

★ So instead of buy, let's say bye to bycatch!

Environmental Devastation

★ Overfishing is the #1 cause of ocean devastation.

★ According to the U.N.'s Food & Agriculture Organization, "Over 70% of the world's fish species are either fully exploited or depleted."

★ The world's fishing fleets are systematically stripping the oceans of sea life, which is rapidly destroying ecosystems that have existed since prehistoric times.

★ Fraud & mislabeling are rampant in the seafood industry.

★ The industry has practices in place to systematically evade efforts to enforce catch limits & human rights standards.

★ Consumers who go out of their way to buy "sustainable" seafood are often purchasing fish from imperiled fisheries.

★ A large meta-study conducted by *Guardian Seascape* in 2021, involving more than 9000 seafood purchases from 30 different countries, identified 40% of samples as mislabeled.

★ Here is a powerful quote from Sea Shepherd Founder, Captain Paul Watson, "*The collapse of ocean bio-diversity and the catastrophic collapse of phytoplankton and zooplankton populations in the sea will cause the collapse of civilization, and most likely the extinction of the human species. And that is why when the ocean dies, we all die!*"

★ According to Captain Watson, the solutions to reversing ocean devastation & the climate crisis are simple ~

1) An end to the ecologically destructive greenhouse-gas-producing animal slaughter industry that emits more greenhouse gases annually than the entire transportation industry.

2) A global moratorium on all industrialized fishing operations.

3) An end to the killing of whales by anyone, anywhere, for any reason.

Farmed Fish

★ Farmed fish do not offer greater sustainability than wild-caught fish.

★ Many farmed fish are genetically modified & fed diets that contain high doses of antibiotics.

★ Intensely crowded undersea cages enable parasites, like sea lice, to thoroughly infest many fish farms.

★ Would you like to live your entire life in a crowded cage & then be killed?

Contamination & Health Risks

★ Eating any kind of fish creates serious health risks.

★ As the world's oceans become increasingly polluted, eating fish becomes fraught with ever-increasing health concerns.

★ According to Dr. Michael Klaper, fish accumulate the pollutants of the modern world in their tissues. Pesticides, herbicides, heavy metals & radioactivity are routinely detected in fish flesh in shockingly high levels, making it the most chemically contaminated of all animal-based foods.

★ Eating fish frequently causes serious biological threats to human health such as fish tapeworms, hepatitis virus, ciguatera toxicity, pathogenic bacteria, etc.

★ To delay spoilage, fish are frequently sprayed with tetracycline & other antibiotics.

★ The concentrated proteins in fish can contribute to the leaching of calcium out of our bones which leads to osteoporosis.

★ Fish can accumulate high levels of mercury & carcinogens like PCBs.

★ An article in *The Telegraph* states that seafood eaters ingest up to 11,000 tiny pieces of plastic every year with dozens of particles becoming embedded in their tissues.

★ Given the volume of non-recycled plastic dumped in our oceans daily, we can only expect seafood contamination risks to grow.

An Ocean of Benefits from Our Beloved Ocean

It appears that many of us take the ocean for granted but without it we could not live. Here are just a few of the ways that we all depend on the ocean to exist ~

★ **The air that we breathe** ~ The ocean produces over half of the world's oxygen & absorbs 50 times more carbon dioxide than our atmosphere.

★ **Fresh water** ~ The oceans of the world play a major role in the fresh water cycle. They form the clouds that bring us rain, which replenish our freshwater supplies.

★ **Climate regulation** ~ The ocean covers 70 % of the Earth's surface & transports heat from the equator to the poles, regulating our climate & weather patterns.

* **Renewable energy** ~ Our oceans provide an invaluable source of renewable, clean energy from tides, ocean currents & powerful waves.

* **Carbon sink** ~ The ocean plays a vital role in the Earth's carbon cycle, removing carbon from the atmosphere & the upper ocean layers. Marine plants also act as carbon sinks by sequestering carbon in seabed sediments. Through this natural storage process, it provides a climate regulation service.

* **Transportation** ~ Ocean-bound shipping accounts for more than 90 percent of global trade.

* **Nutrition & Medicine** ~ Marine plants such as sea grasses, algae & sea vegetables provide valuable nutrition & have medicinal properties.

* **Recreation & Rejuvenation** ~ The ocean provides us with the opportunity for many unique activities such as swimming, diving, snorkeling, surfing, paddle boarding, kite surfing, parasailing, canoeing, kayaking, sailing, whale watching & of course, mermaiding! We all know how taking a walk on the beach & spending time at the seaside can be so healing & uplifting for mind, body & soul!

The intricate workings that keep the ocean & our planet in a perfect symbiotic balance, are reaching their tipping point. Ocean devastation results in human devastation. Overfishing is the #1 cause of ocean devastation. It is based on supply & demand, so by eliminating our consumption of fish, we can help our beloved oceans to restore & renew.

Omega 3 Fatty Acids

* Research indicates that fish offer excellent sources of omega 3s, DHA & EPA.

* These fat molecules are associated with better brain health.

* Fortunately, there are rich vegan sources of these fats without ingesting the biochemistry of terror, which is released when torturing & killing living beings and without devastating our oceans.

* Chia seeds are full of this fat. You can improve your intake of omega 3 by incorporating chia seeds into your daily diet. Chia seeds are great in cereal, mixed into plant milk, in chia pudding or used as an egg-replacer. Just a couple teaspoons a day will boost your intake to levels that experts recommend.

* Including flax seeds & hemp seeds in your diet is also highly beneficial. Each tablespoon of ground flaxseed contains about 1.8 grams of plant omega-3s & 1 ounce (28 grams) of hemp seeds contains 6,000 mg of ALA omega-3 fatty acids, or 375–545% of the daily recommended intake.

* Grinding your seeds will significantly increase your body's absorption of omega 3s.

* Your body can convert omega 3 into DHA & EPA which are two important brain nutrients.

* People vary widely in their ability to create DHA & EPA from omega 3, so you might want to consider taking vegan supplements.

★ A common misconception is that fish products are the only source of these two substances. Fortunately, you can purchase vegan supplements that are derived from algae & contain both DHA & EPA.

★ Since the fish get these nutrients from algae, you can get it directly from algae & thereby cut out the middle man!

★ Vegan omega 3 supplements are also much less likely than fish-derived supplements to contain appreciable amounts of mercury, plastics & other contaminants.

★ Some popular vegan brands are DEVA Amala Vegan, Ovega-3 & Dr. Fuhrman's DHA & EPA Purity.

Vegan Fish Products & Recipes

Eliminating fish & shrimp from your diet is easier today than ever before. There are many vegan products that do a fantastic job of capturing the tastes & textures of seafood such as ~

★ Gardein ~ Golden Fishless Fillet & Crabless Cakes

★ Sophies Kitchen ~ Vegan Crab Cakes, Fish Fillet, Shrimp, Scallops, Smoked Salmon & Toona

★ Good Catch Foods ~ Fish Burgers, Fish Cakes, Crab Cakes & 3 varieties of vegan tuna.

★ You can even buy a cookbook devoted entirely to vegan seafood recipes entitled, *Everything That Used to Have Fish is Now Vegan.*

★ Now is a great time to eliminate seafood from your diet. As it is said so well on *vegan.com*, *"The reasons have never been so compelling & the alternatives have never been so plentiful!"*

★ I highly recommend the documentary, *Seapiracy*, which is available on Netflix, to further elaborate on this topic.

How to Transition to a Plant-Based Diet with Ease, Grace & Joy

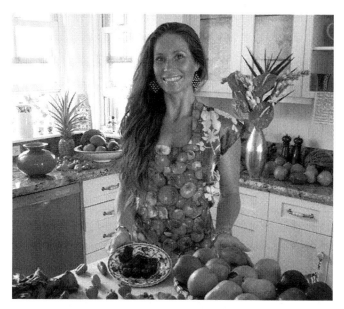

One of my precious vegan kindred Spirits, Brook Le'amohala

"Always be the vegan that you would've wanted to meet before you were vegan yourself."
- Vegan Tweeter

★ If you are a non-vegetarian, become a vegetarian.
  If you are a vegetarian, become a vegan.
  If you are a vegan, become a thriving vegan & an effective vegan educator!

★ Regarding becoming a vegan educator, sometimes it can feel like a daunting task, because there is so much ignorance & cruelty in this world.

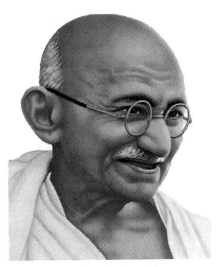
Mahatma Gandhi

"Many people, especially ignorant people, want to punish you for speaking the truth, for being correct, for being you. Never apologize for being correct, or for being years ahead of your time. If you're right & you know it, speak your mind. Even if you are a minority of one, the truth is still the truth."
- Mahatma Gandhi

This is a good time to draw inspiration from Helen Keller, who said, *"I am only one, but still I am one. I cannot do everything, but still I can do something. I will not refuse to do the something I can do."*

Also from Yogi Bhajan, who said, *"If you want to learn something, read about it. If you want to understand something, write about it. If you want to master something, teach it."*

"Never be afraid to raise your voice for honesty, truth & compassion against injustice, lying & greed. If people all over the world would do it, it would change the earth."
- William Faulkner

And in this case, **save** the Earth! Please wake up from this cultural trance!

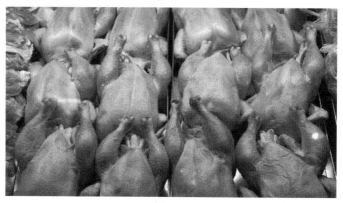

"To ignore evil is to become an accomplice to it."
- Dr. Martin Luther King Jr.

"I was not born to fit into this world. I was born to create a new one." - StarShine Path-to-Truth

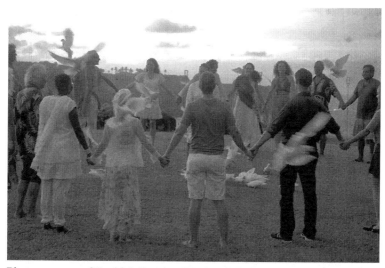

Photo courtesy of Fredrick Swaroop Honig ~ TheGardens.org. Maui, Hawaii

"It is only with love & compassion that we can begin to mend what is broken in this world." - Dr. Steve Maraboli

"Don't worry if you are making waves simply by being yourself. The Moon does it all of the time!" - Scott Stabile

A Few Practical, Fun & Easy Tips

"An ounce of practice is worth more than a ton of theory."
- Master Sivananda, MD

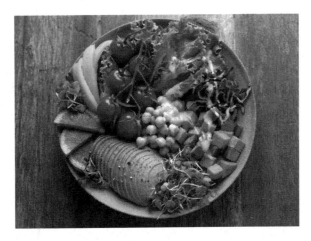

★ Explore countless delicious vegan recipes from YouTube, books, websites, apps & friends.

★ Make vegan versions of your favorite meals.

★ Visit your local health food store & check out vegan options.

★ Try some tasty meat-free & dairy-free products.

★ Discover some vegan convenience foods.

★ Search online for vegan-friendly restaurants & stores near you.

★ Join a vegan meet-up group.

★ Ask people what is their favorite vegan go-to meal.

★ Engage family members & friends to co-create a vegan meal.

★ Host a vegan potluck.

★ Explore vegan international cuisine.

★ Host a vegan movie night with popcorn & discuss afterwards.

★ Become a vegan mentor.

★ Invest in vegan businesses.

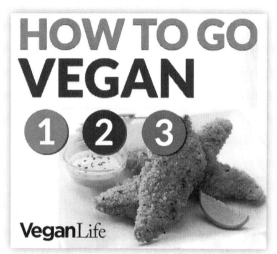

How to go vegan in three simple steps ~
①. What to buy. ②. What to make. ③. Where to eat.

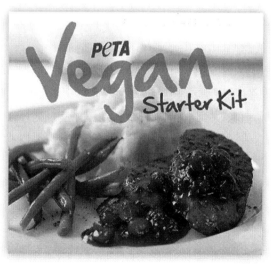

PETA Vegan Starter Kit http://features.peta.org/how-to-go-vegan

Check out the Resource Pages at the end of this book for some more great recommendations!

Seven Guidelines for Optimum Nutrition

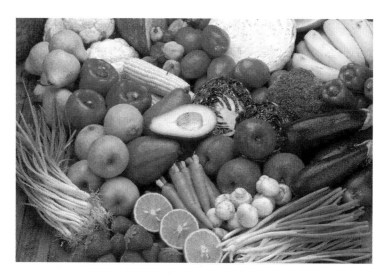

"Good nutrition will prevent 95% of all disease."
- Linus Pauling, Nobel Peace Prize Laureate

1) Cruelty-free

Select a compassionate, whole foods plant-based diet, as much as possible.

2) Straight-from-the source, organic & GMO free

This means, as much as possible, to eat food the way that nature brings it, rather than processed food. For example ~ choose potatoes, rather than potato chips; corn, rather than corn chips; rice, rather than rice cakes, etc.

As my Beloved Gurudev, Sri Swami Satchidananda said, *"The same One who made the colon made the apple, not the apple pie."*

Whole food in its natural state has its *prana* (life force energy), intelligence, fiber, vitamins, minerals, nutrients, & so on. When food is processed, it becomes devitalized, so choose wisely. Eating organic food that is free of toxic chemicals is healthier for your body temple, as well as for the body temple of our precious Mother Earth.

3) Mindfulness

Be present with your food! Give your full loving attention to preparing & chewing your food.

See if you can slow down your eating process & really merge your attention with every taste, texture, pore & aspect of your food.

Avoid doing other activities while you are eating so that you can really focus on your food.

Chew thoroughly until your food is liquefied—before swallowing & reaching for more.

By consciously engaging all of your senses—seeing, smelling, touching, hearing & tasting—in the eating process, you will enjoy your food more & feel more satisfied. What a pleasurable way to develop & practice mindfulness!

4) Quantity ~ Moderation

Eating slowly & mindfully helps with cultivating the habit of moderation. Research has shown that it takes approximately 20 minutes from the time you start eating for your brain to send out signals of fullness.

It is beneficial to set a timer for 20 minutes & slow down your eating process, so that your brain has enough time to get the message that you are satiated.

Then, you will be less likely to reach for seconds & you will find yourself eating more moderately.

Engaging in a cleanse, a mono diet, or a liquid diet & fasting periodically are also beneficial ways to develop the practice of eating moderately.

These practices help to interrupt addictive eating patterns & give us the opportunity to re-enter our relationship with food in a more conscious & moderate way.

5) Timing

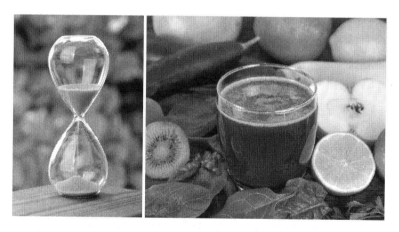

Avoid eating, whenever possible, for two hours before practicing *Hatha Yoga* (physical postures), *pranayama* (breathing practices), exercise, massage & sleep.

There are only about 8 pints of blood in the body & it has its priority systems. If the blood is being called to the limbs, it detracts from digestion, so it is best not to do strenuous exercise right after eating.

If you avoid eating before receiving a therapeutic massage, the blood that would have gone into digestion is free to go into healing your body temple.

If you avoid eating before sleep, the blood that would go into digestion is free to do repair & maintenance while you sleep. This results in waking up feeling more refreshed & with a higher level of wellbeing.

6) Gratitude

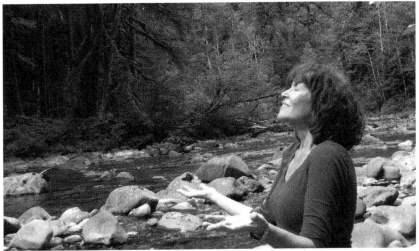

Archangel Rebecca McLean ~ Photo courtesy of Roger Jahnke

Pause for a prayer that is meaningful to you & tune into the feeling of gratitude before eating.

Research has shown that when we stop to pray before eating, digestive enzymes are released which improve digestion, assimilation & elimination.

It is beautiful to note the complementary relationship here, between the physical & the metaphysical.

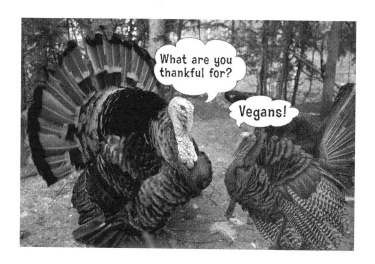

7) Dedication

Use the life force energy from the food, to love & serve, in whatever way is your unique calling.

This way we are not debtors to nature; but, rather, we are just recycling the energy.

A carrot, on its own, may not be able to do much; but, through you, a lot can be achieved.

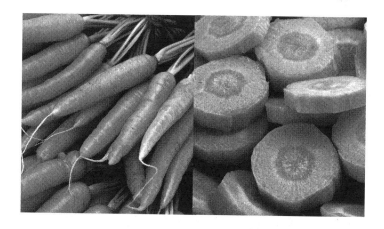

Being vegan is the kind choice for the animals, the environment & for your own health.

Being kind is the essence underlying every Spiritual path.

"Every thought you produce, anything you say, any action you do, it bears your signature."
- Thich Nhat Hanh

What do you want your Soul signature to be?

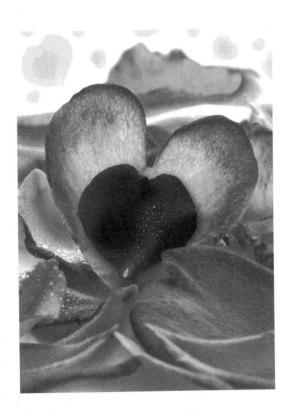

Cleansing Diet

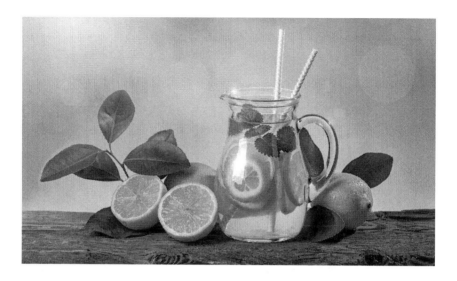

"Cleanliness is next to Godliness!"

What we eat has a huge impact on how we feel!

If you want to feel your best & have your best to give, I highly recommend having an organic, as much as possible, whole food plant-based diet, all year round.

In addition to that, I suggest doing a cleanse four times per year.

No matter how diligent we are with our dietary choices, there are still other factors at play that affect our wellbeing such as toxic chemicals in the environment, GMOs that we may not even be aware of, harmful electronic emissions, stress & pollution.

This all adds up to it being a good idea to do a cleanse, to give your organs a break, to drop a few excess pounds that may have crept up on you & to give your body temple a chance to rejuvenate itself.

Remember, there are about 8 pints of blood in the body. If it is not going into digesting food, it is free to do repair & maintenance, which results in a higher level of wellness.

Here are a few good reasons to do a cleanse ~

★ Shed a few extra pounds.

★ Feel & look our best.

★ By consciously eating more straight-from-the-source food, we have more energy & clarity to work on our projects.

★ Our seeing, hearing, smelling, tasting & feeling become more acute.

★ Aches & pains disappear.

★ We feel more limber in our body temples, in our Yoga practice & in our exercise routines.

★ We go deeper in meditation.

★ If you do a cleanse right before your birthday, you can usher in each new year on the best possible note. This sets a good tone for the whole year.

★ When we feel our best, we have better energy to share with others.

★ When we feel our best, we have higher self-esteem & become positive role models for others.

★ Those who are older can serve as living examples by being in good shape. This contributes to a new paradigm for graceful eldering.

★ When we eat more consciously, we develop more self-mastery. This allows us to access higher dimensions of consciousness, which feels sublime!

★ When we feel light, it is easier to be the light & to delight one & all!

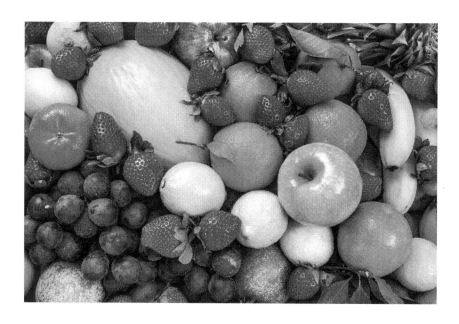

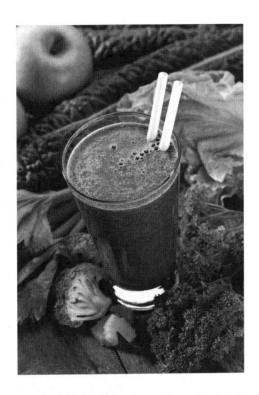

A few options to consider for cleansing & lightening up include ~

★ Fasting on water

★ Liquid diet ~ herbal teas, vegetable broth, fruit & vegetable juices

★ Smoothies

★ Blended soups

★ Mono diet

★ Straight-from-the-source diet

Straight-from-the-source diet means eating food the way nature brings it, rather than processed foods.

In the summer time, I love to do a cleanse eating just watermelon for a few days!

Another option for a cleanse is to eat primarily raw fruits, vegetables & sprouts.

In other cleanses, I have included a small amount of raw seeds & nuts such as sunflower, pumpkin, hemp, cashews, almonds, walnuts, hazelnuts, macadamia nuts & pistachios.

It is a good practice to get into the rhythm of choosing one day per week to do a liquid diet or a cleansing diet that is high in raw fruits & vegetables. This is a consistent & gentle way to give your body temple a chance to cleanse & rejuvenate which results in a higher level of wellbeing on all levels!

Feel Great at Your Ideal Weight

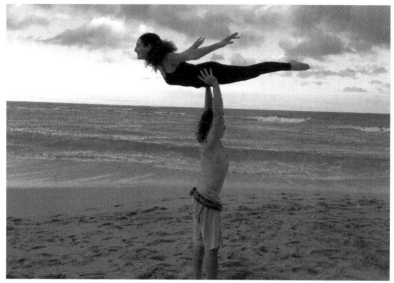

Meenakshi Angel Honig ~ Flying Yoga

"You can kiss your weight concerns goodbye because if you eat a whole foods, unprocessed plant-based diet in moderation, your weight will take care of itself."
- Meenakshi Angel Honig

As I mentioned, vegans are on the average 20 pounds lighter that their non-vegan counterparts.

An estimated 45 million Americans go on a diet each year & Americans spend $33 billion each year on weight loss products.

This, my friends, can be radically simplified! Not only can you live in accordance with your values of lovingkindness & compassion but you can also save money with this simple & highly effective weight management approach!

If you eat a whole foods unprocessed plant-based diet, in moderation, your weight will automatically normalize itself & come to the weight that is ideal for your body type. In the Yoga way of thinking, there are 3 different body types; kapha, pita & vata. Some body types are naturally like a pumpkin, others like a zucchini & others like a string bean. Eating a whole foods vegan diet will not make a pumpkin into a string bean. It will, however, make each body type the healthiest version of itself.

I do want to emphasize a *whole foods* vegan diet as opposed to a *junk food* vegan diet. French fries cooked in oil, soft drinks & Oreo cookies are vegan but that does not constitute a healthy diet. Whole foods means foods in their natural state, as much as possible, such as whole grains, legumes, fresh vegetables, fruits, sprouts, nuts & seeds in moderation.

You can combine these whole foods in creative ways that are incredibly delicious & nutritious. This is not a deprivation; it is a higher choice!

Choosing a whole foods plant-based diet, along with moderate exercise that you enjoy, Yoga, breathing practices, stress management, meditation, good rest & dedicating your life to a noble purpose that is greater than yourself are the pillars of radiant health & wellbeing.

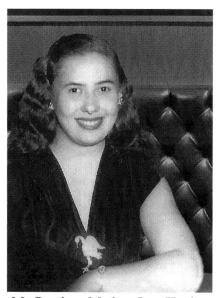

My Precious Mother, Jean Honig

When I was growing up, my dear precious Mother was very devoted to her family. She didn't take the time to exercise, practice Hatha Yoga, eat carefully, or implement other self-care techniques. Her main exercise was going up & down the steps to do the laundry & taking care of her five children, her husband, my grandmother & everyone who was blessed to know her.

While she was very dedicated to taking the best care of others, she did not take the best care of herself. Consequently, she was overweight. I saw & felt how much pain this caused her, both physically & emotionally.

I made an inner commitment to myself that I would never let myself get overweight, because I did not want to have to deal with that kind of pain, if I could avoid it.

So, I created a system for myself that has served me very well & has also served countless students & clients of mine over many years. I would like to share it with you, with the hopes that it will serve you, as well!

I decided to use a scale as a healthy barometer to keep myself on track. I got clear on a range of weight that felt right for me.

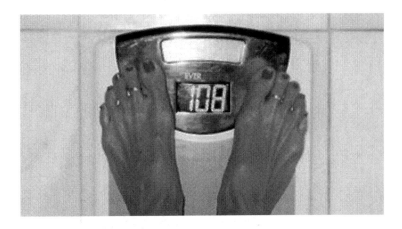

I decided that under 110 was excellent; because I feel my absolute best & on pitch with the entire Universe when my body temple weights 108 pounds!

Between 110 & 115 is good.

Between 115 & 120 is acceptable, but over 120 is not acceptable for me.

So, I weigh in regularly & if I see that my weight is creeping up, I go on a cleanse to get it back into the zone that feels best to me.

It is sooooo much better & easier to nip it in the bud than to let it get out of control!

According to the *National Health & Nutrition Examination Survey*, more than two out of three adults in the U.S. are considered to be overweight or obese.

About one-third of children & adolescents, ages 6 to 19, are considered to be overweight or obese.

Being overweight & obese are both risk factors for type-2 diabetes, heart disease, high blood pressure, osteoarthritis, cancer, strokes & a host of other health problems.

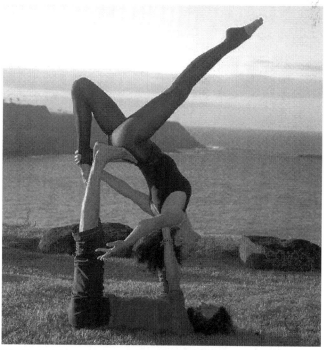

Meenakshi Angel Honig & Allowah Lani ~ Flying Yoga
Photo by Fredrick Swaroop Honig

Food is one of the most abused anxiety drugs & exercise is one of the most underutilized antidepressants!

One of the many valuable things that I learned from Dr. Sandra Amrita McLanahan, a medical doctor who received additional training from my beloved teacher, Swami Satchidananda, is that whatever we eat, we crave.

Therefore, if you decide what you want to crave, such as fruit, vegetables, whole grains, legumes, nuts, seeds & sprouts, you can then reverse engineer & start eating those foods. In a very short amount of time, it is those exact foods that you will crave! So, it's easy to set yourself up to succeed!

I encourage you to make a list of the reasons why it would be beneficial for you to do a cleanse for your body temple.

Then, decide on a range of weight that feels good to you, as I have described. Weigh in regularly & keep yourself in the weight zone where you feel your best & thrive!

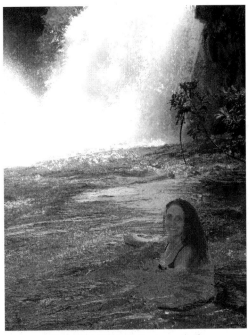

Photo by Brook Le'amohala

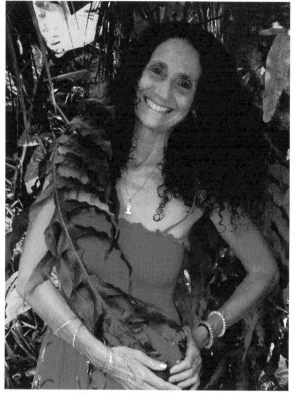
Photo by Kati Alexandra

If you would like some coaching & support with this, please feel welcome to contact me at www.AngelYoga.com.

Graceful Eldering

"May the rest of your life be the best of your life!"

Another good reason to choose a plant-based diet is to embody & promote graceful eldering.

Given that we live in a culture that gives disproportional emphasis to having a youthful appearance, rather than honoring the beauty in all stages of life, many people fall prey to invasive & expensive procedures, in an attempt to keep up with an illusory youthful image that is propagated by the media.

According to the annual plastic surgery procedural statistics, there were 17.5 million surgical cosmetic procedures performed in the USA in 2017, a 2% increase over 2016. In 2018, the global anti-aging market was estimated to be worth about 50.2 billion dollars. The anti-aging market is estimated to see a compound annual growth rate of 5.7 % between 2018 & 2023.

My beloved teacher, Swami Satchidananda, said, *"Cultivate the cosmic beauty, not the cosmetic beauty."*

A vegan diet is rich in antioxidants & phytonutrients. Phytochemicals, also called phytonutrients, are naturally occurring compounds in plant foods such as fruits, vegetables, whole grains, beans, nuts & seeds. In laboratory studies, many phytochemicals act as antioxidants, neutralizing free radicals & removing their power to create damage. Phytochemicals have protective qualities for human health which support a more youthful appearance.

According to Nathalie Rhone, MS, RDN, CDN, here are ten foods that are jam-packed with nutrients to promote glowing skin & promote radiant wellbeing ~

1) Watercress
2) Red bell pepper
3) Papaya
4) Blueberries
5) Broccoli
6) Spinach
7) Nuts
8) Avocado
9) Sweet potatoes
10) Pomegranate seeds

Choose fruits & vegetables that are deep in color. The rich shades are usually a sign of stronger radical fighting abilities to keep your skin healthy & vibrant. The more colors of the rainbow that you include on your plate, the better.

I attribute feeling great at my ideal weight & graceful eldering to an unprocessed whole foods vegan diet along with other healthy lifestyle choices such as alignment with Divine benevolence, love, yoga, meditation, breathing practices, prayer, walking & swimming in nature, gratitude & meaningful service.

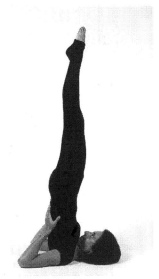
Angel at 30

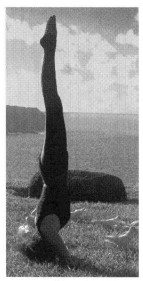
Angel at 60

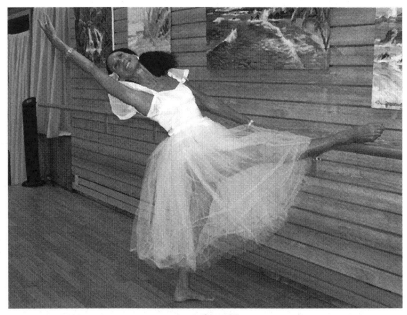
Angel at 65

Due to the glory of Yoga & an unprocessed whole foods vegan diet, I am astounded & grateful that at age 65, I can fit into the ***exact*** ballet costume that I wore at age 14, without ***any*** alteration!

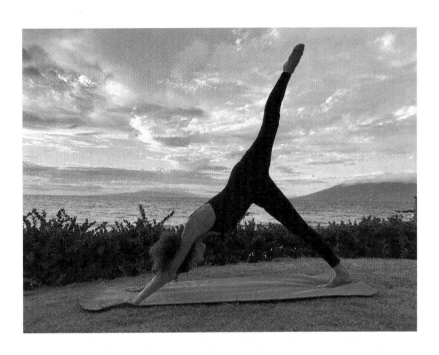

Angel at age 67

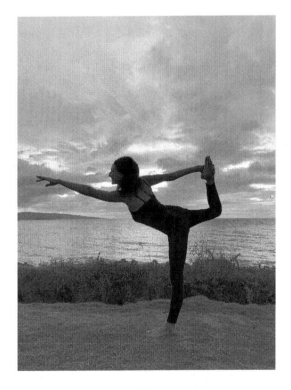

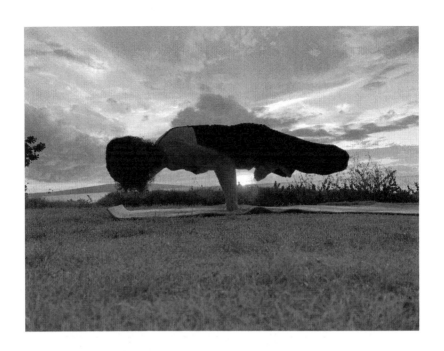

Photos by of Julie Stuehser

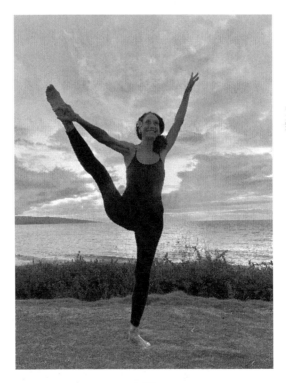

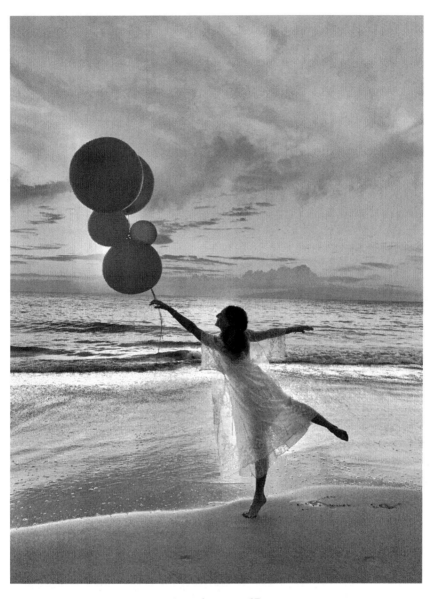

Angel at age 67

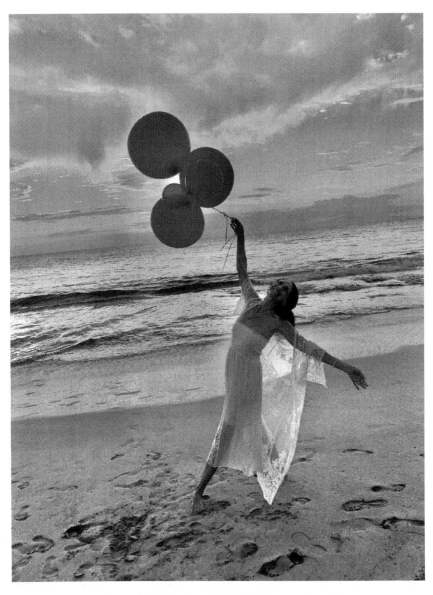

Photos by of Julie Stuehser

Regardless of what age you are, if you would like to feel your best, look your best, be your best & give your best, wouldn't this be a great time to ***go vegan!***

Say NO to GMO

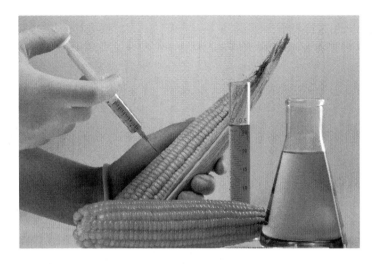

"How could we have ever believed that it was a good idea to grow our food with poisons?"
- Jane Goodall

Here are some compelling reasons from Jeffrey Smith, author of Genetic Roulette, to clear your life & this world of GMOs. (Genetically Modified Organisms)

★ GMOs carry significant health dangers.

★ Releasing GMOs outdoors leads to irreversible contamination of the ecosystem.

★ The use of the herbicide Roundup is dramatically increased with GM Roundup Ready crops. This negatively affects human, animal, plant & environmental health.

★ The process of genetic engineering is imprecise, fraught with unpredictable side effects & is based on obsolete assumptions.

★ The industry-funded research is superficial & largely rigged to avoid finding problems. Independent scientists who discover problems are attacked & media seeking to expose these problems are censored.

★ GMOs lead to environmental problems such as loss of bio-diversity & harm to birds, bees, insects & soil ecology.

★ GMOs do not help feed the world but, rather, work against that goal.

Whereas, going

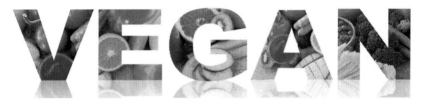

significantly contributes to ending starvation worldwide!

If you care about having the right to eat organic food made by nature, without toxic chemicals, please view this free movie, *Seeds of Death*, on YouTube & share it widely, so that every citizen of planet Earth can make an informed choice!

www.youtube.com/watch?v=J4Z1Bu-XAm0

Or watch the DVD entitled, *Genetic Roulette: The Gamble of Our Lives* by Jeffrey Smith.

"To pretend that poison is not poison, is poison itself."
- Dr. Martin Luther King, Jr.

By avoiding GMOs, you can help to generate the tipping point of consumer rejection of this toxicity.

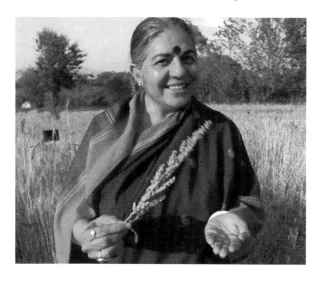

As Vandana Shiva said so clearly,

"If they control seed, they control food. They know it. It's strategic. It's more powerful than bombs & it's more powerful than guns. This is the best way to control the populations of the world."

If you want to feel your best, eat organic!

By choosing organic, we contribute to freeing animals, wildlife & our precious Mother Earth from GMOs & from the toxic chemicals that accompany them!

To Bee or Not to Bee

"If the bee disappeared off the face of the earth, man would only have four years left to live."
- Maurice Maeterlinck

* Bees are widely considered to be one of the most important species on the planet.

* According to livekindly.com, approximately 250,000 species of flowering plants rely on bees for pollination.

* Bees are responsible for the pollination of over **90%** of the plants that we eat.

* Without bees, fruit & vegetable stocks would deplete.

* There are 20,000 different types of bees in the world but only one kind makes honey & that is the honeybee. *Female* "worker" bees produce honey from pollen & nectar that they collect from plants on their fuzzy bodies while pollinating. They then store the honey in honeycombs made of wax inside their nest.

* Male bees, or drones, don't do any work. They make up roughly 10% of the colony's population & they spend their whole lives eating honey & waiting for the opportunity to mate.

* It takes more than 550 bees to gather 1 pound of honey from roughly 2 million flowers, according to the Apex Bee Company.

* Bees will fly 55,000 miles to make a gallon of honey.

* The average bee will make only 1/12 of a teaspoon of honey in her life & bees rely on this as their primary food source.

* Bees are classified as both insects & animals. They are intelligent & have a complex communication system.

An article on factory farming bees, presented by *ThinkDifferentlyAboutSheep.weebly.com*, heightened my awareness about how bees are manipulated worldwide to produce many products for human use, such as honey, beeswax, propolis, bee pollen, royal jelly & venom.

Many people think that bees make honey for our use, just as many believe that cows make milk for humans. Cow's milk is meant to feed baby calves, just as human milk is meant to feed baby humans & honey is meant to feed bees. Large scale bee keepers steal all their honey & feed the colony with sugar syrup or corn syrup.

I feel that we have a lot to learn from bees & I am inspired by this quote from Thomas Young, *"Their loyalty and attachment to their queen cannot be surpassed: no distress or extremity is able to overcome it. Nor is their patriotism inferior to their loyalty. Every private interest and every appetite seems to centre, or rather to be lost, in a zeal for the public good. In laboring for this they wear out their little lives, which they are ready every moment to sacrifice in its defense. Each restrains its own appetite in order to bring the greatest possible addition to the common stock of honey; and when the cells are once closed up, it does not presume to break one of them open, unless urged by absolute necessity, and even then exhibits a pattern of frugality and temperance: but if the public stores be attacked, no inequality of strength or size will deter it from assaulting the aggressor."*

★ Many vegans do not eat honey so as not to harm bees. They believe that exploiting bees for their labor & harvesting their energy source is immoral. They point out that large-scale beekeeping operations harm & kill bees.

★ Because bees are seen flying free, people may not realize that they are subjected to the cruelties of the animal farming industry. Bees from commercial operations have to endure routine examination, handling, artificial feeding regimes, drug & pesticide treatment, genetic manipulation, artificial insemination, transportation (by air, rail & road) & slaughter.

★ Bees are hardworking animals who deserve to "bee" free & keep the honey for which they work so diligently. Stealing products from them is a form of exploitation that can be easily avoided.

★ Honey can be replaced by rice syrup, barley malt, maple syrup, molasses, sorghum, coconut syrup or fruit concentrates. I personally use blended dates in place of honey.

★ Thankfully for honey-lovers, there are plenty of vegan alternatives available such as *Bee Free Honee*, which makes an ethical honey out of organic apples.

★ *D'vash Organics* is the producer of what it claims is the world's first sweet potato honey.

★ So why not be sweet & let the bees be?

* There are, however, some devoted vegans & vegan advocates, such as my brother Swaroop, who feel that bees can thrive with compassionate organic bee keepers. He feels that bees are better off in human luxury hive arrangements than having to deal with rotten logs, rain storms & attacks from bears & ants.

* Swaroop believes that it is necessary to have bee keepers who are dedicated to the wellbeing of their bees. He asserts that without bee keepers watching out for the health of their bees, bees would be at the peril of nature which is not easy for bees these days.

* Swaroop is an advocate of ingesting raw, local, organic, compassionately-sourced honey to increase immunity as well as many other health benefits.

* Although I personally do not use honey, beeswax, propolis, royal jelly & other products that come from bees, when it comes to honey that is sourced from careful & compassionate organic bee keepers, as opposed to factory farmed bees in commercial operations, I encourage you to put on your critical thinking cap, tune into your heart, your conscience & do a gut check to discover what resonates as true for you.

Break Up with Non-Vegan Makeup!

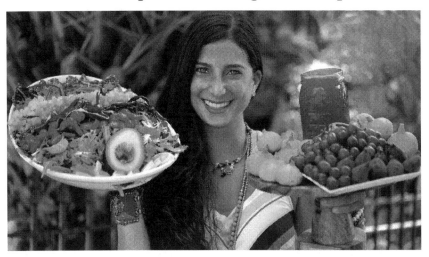

A few years ago, I saw a life-changing video by Fully Raw Kristina. Fully Raw Kristina is a bright light, who has a YouTube channel that I highly recommend for fantastic raw vegan recipes that are beautifully presented! She also addresses many other vegan topics in her video offerings.

In this particular video, Kristina was quoting research from an article on PETA's website about what goes into conventional lipstick, blush, cosmetics & other beauty products.

I was shocked to hear Kristina say that the red pigment commonly used in these products is derived from the guts of thousands of ground up beetles! In fact, it takes up to 70,000 beetles to make one pound of dye.

So, when you are applying conventional lipstick, you are smearing the insides of thousands of dead insects on your lips! Imagine kissing someone with this on your lips or eating food & swallowing some of it. Yikes! (I know this information may be hard to swallow!)

As my beloved teacher, Swami Satchidananda, said, *"When you realize you are holding a cobra snake, drop it!"*

So, I immediately dropped using conventional lipstick & replaced it with *100% Pure* lipstick. This conscious company makes strictly vegan make-up that is derived from fruit pigments, such as pomegranate, instead of crushed insects.

If you would like to determine if crushed beetles are in your lipstick, simply look for these ingredients: "CI 75470," "cochineal extract," "crimson lake," "natural red 4," or "carmine."

These ingredients may also be found in ~
★ Cosmetics
★ Shampoos
★ Red applesauce
★ Other foods including red lollipops, yogurt, drinks & food coloring

If you find this hard to believe, check it out for yourself. Here is a link to the article from PETA that Kristina was quoting ~
www.peta.org/living/personal-care-fashion/carmine-makeup/

There are also a host of other cruel & disgusting ingredients contained in everyday beauty care & household items. If people really realized what goes into these products, they would be repulsed. Therefore, many manufacturers disguise the ingredients with deceptive terms so that very few people know what they actually mean & how they are sourced.

Here are a few common examples of these ingredients & *who* & *what* they are made of ~

★ Gelatin or Collagen - Pigs' & cows' skin & bones

★ Keratin - Ground up hooves or feathers

★ Helix aspersa muller glycoconjugates or snail cream - Snail slime

★ Afterbirth, placental polypeptide protein or placenta - Placenta taken from the uterus of slaughtered animals

★ Cat Glandular Secretion - Secretion painfully scraped from a gland very near the genital organs of civet cats

★ Musk Oil - Secretion that's painfully obtained from musk deer, beaver, muskrat, civet cat & otter genitals

★ Ambergris - Whale vomit

★ Shark Liver Oil or Squalene - Oil from the liver of sharks

★ Mink Oil - Oil taken from the fat of slaughtered minks

★ Mayonnaise or Eggs - Mayonnaise is made with eggs, which result from chicken menstruation

★ Urea or Carbamide - Animal urine

★ Sodium tallowate, tallowate, sodium taloate - Cow or sheep lard

★ Lanolin, aliphatic alcohols, cholesterin, isopropyl lanolate, laneth, Lanogene, lanolin alcohols, lanosterol, sterols, or triterpene alcohols - Lanolin is the natural grease that coats sheep's wool to keep the animals dry & protect their skin.

To see a more complete list please check out PETA's Animal Derived Ingredient List ~
www.peta.org/living/food/animal-ingredients-list/

By being informed, we can make more discerning, compassionate & healthy choices!

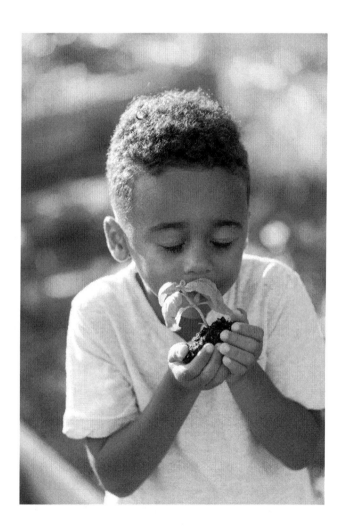

Evolution of a Soul

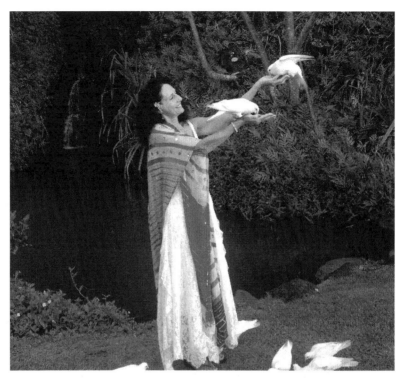

"We do the best we can with what we know & when we know better, we do better."
- Maya Angelou

While there are countless wonderful vegan cookbooks, vegan YouTube channels, plant-based meats & dairy substitutes readily available, I personally eat only ***unprocessed or minimally processed*** vegan food for two main reasons.

1) As I mentioned earlier, the same/sane One who made the colon, made the apple, not the apple pie. Food is information & whole food transmits wholeness. When we eat foods, as much as possible, in their natural state the way nature brings them, they have their wholeness, fiber, intelligence, vitamins, minerals, nutrients & vitality.

They are in the right proportion that was intended by our great Creator for our body temples. Whenever we process food, we devitalize it & take it out of proportion which is not optimal for our digestion, assimilation & elimination. So, eating whole organic food, as much as possible, is the healthiest choice for our body temples as well as for our precious Mother Earth.

2) It was brought to my attention in a pivotal, life-changing conversation that I had with Ryan Earhart, who is the owner of Okoa Farms on Maui & has been involved in the food industry for decades, that all processed food is inadvertently ground up with insect fragments & a host of other disgusting debris such as mold, rodent hair & excreta.

When Ryan told me this, I was in a state of shock & disbelief, so he gave me this explanation. He said, *"When someone is harvesting tomatoes, whether they be organic or commercial, they pick the tomatoes & put them in a truck. The truck may be in the sun all day while they are harvesting other tomatoes. During this time there may be bugs, worms, mites & rodents visiting these tomatoes. Do you think they hire someone to pick out every fruit fly that lands in that truck?"*

He then went on to explain that the truck of tomatoes is then taken to a plant where the tomatoes are processed & that a significant amount of that debris gets ground up into your tomato sauce.

When I was in a state of further shock & disbelief, Ryan said, *"If you don't believe me, just go to the FDA website & look up their "Food Defect Levels Handbook" & you will see in black & white the amounts of filth that is allowable in the everyday food that we eat."*

I did go to the FDA website & sure enough everything that Ryan shared with me was accurate. Here is the link for the *FDA Food Defect Levels Handbook* so that you can see for yourself!

www.fda.gov/food/ingredients-additives-gras-packaging-guidance-documents-regulatory-information/food-defect-levels-handbook

Because the thought of eating cockroaches & rodent excreta is disgusting to me, to put it mildly, I decided to do an experiment to see if I could live in this society without eating processed food.

I didn't know even one single other person who was eating this way, so I had to think it through for myself. First, I made a list of all the food that I could eat because I could wash it & see clearly that it was not ground up with this disgusting debris.

On my list I wrote ~
- Fruits
- Vegetables
- Whole Grains
- Whole legumes
- Seeds
- Nuts
- Sprouts
- Pink Himalayan salt crystals
- Fresh Herbs

Then I called my precious BFF & purpose partner, Rebecca McLean, who is the supreme coach of coaches, angel of angels & developer of the *Circle of Life Health & Wellness Coaching Process*™.

I explained the whole life-changing situation to her & asked for her support in my doing a one-month experiment to see if I could live in this culture without eating processed foods.

With her support, I embarked on the experiment. Although it has required some significant adjustments, I found a way to make it work & have never looked back. In fact, I keep discovering & creating ever-new *unprocessed* luscious recipes!

I became a vegetarian when I was around 11 years old. I was repulsed when I realized that meat came from killing animals. This was before computers & the internet; before kids had access to massive information instantly. I did not know even one single vegetarian at that time. I became the first vegetarian that I ever met!

Then, like most people at that time, I was under the illusion that cows were happily grazing in green pastures & lovingly gave their milk to caregivers who knew them by name & sang to them. I did not know about the horrific suffering that is inflicted on dairy cows to force them to lactate continuously & then steal the milk that was intended for their calves.

Then when John Robbin's book entitled, *Diet for a New America* came out in 1987, a friend of mine read it. He was so deeply moved by the book that he created a handout that summarized the key points. My friend gave me the handout to read & by the time I finished reading it, I shifted from being a vegetarian to a vegan. Up until that time I did not know the cruel torture that cows are forced to endure for humans to have milk & milk products. The second that I was informed, I became a vegan for life & that was over 30 years ago.

I never even read the book, which just goes to show that every effort toward vegan advocacy is valuable because we never know what is going to touch who & when.

This is why I am writing this book, because I know that when people find out what is really going on behind closed doors, they make new more informed, compassionate choices.

As Paul McCartney said, *"If slaughter houses had glass walls, everyone would be a vegetarian."* I take that a step farther & say that if everyone would go to a factory farm, they would be a vegan!

It is my sincere hope & prayer that this book will land in the lap or laptop of someone who will be inspired by reading this this, just as I was inspired by reading the handout based on a *Diet for a New America*, to Go Vegan!

"When we know better, we do better!"
- Maya Angelou

Setting Yourself Up to Succeed
This is not a diet; this is a lifestyle

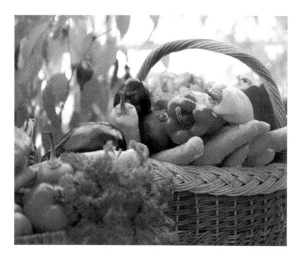

"Fortune favors the prepared."
- Louis Pasteur

Now that you have read and hopefully taken to heart my *10 Compelling Reasons to Choose a Plant-based Diet*, let's move from the **why to the how**.

Eating healthy food is not a diet, it is a lifestyle. It is a state of consciousness based on living in alignment with your values. *"First you form your habits, then your habits form you!"*

Master Sivananda, who was a medical doctor & one of the greatest enlightened Yoga masters who ever walked on planet Earth, said, *"Your thoughts affect your words, your words affect your actions, your actions affect your habits, your habits affect your character & your character affects your destiny."*

So, it is through your thoughts, words & actions that you can create a healthy or unhealthy destiny or outcome. The choice is yours, so choose the good ones!

Setting Yourself Up to Succeed

Whenever you want to be successful in upgrading your lifestyle habits, it is very helpful to have the right accoutrements to support your new venture.

For example, if you want to start jogging, it is helpful to get the appropriate running shoes, (unless you jog barefoot on the beach :)) and if you want to go camping it is useful to get a backpack & sleeping bag, etc. Similarly, if you want to eat healthy food, it is very helpful to have a few items to set yourself up to succeed.

I love this quote ~ *"If you fail to plan, plan to fail."*

Here are a few items that I use on a daily basis. I always have some healthy food & beverages with me. When you are prepared with healthy food options, you will be much less likely to reach for junk food when you need a pick-me-up.

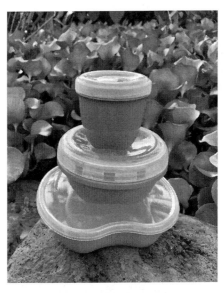

1) Eco-friendly Plastic Containers ~ 3 sizes

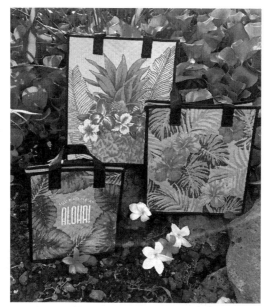

Photos by Julie Stuehser

2) Thermal Bags ~ 3 sizes

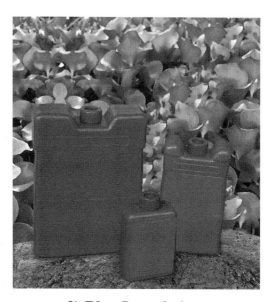

3) Blue Ice ~ 3 sizes

When I leave the house, I take these items with me so that I am well prepared regardless of what the day brings.

1) My glass water bottle with the reusable straw is filled with my special ginger/turmeric tea that I put in the cup holder in my Angelmobile, for when I am driving.
(Tea recipe is on page 305.)

2) The other glass water bottle with the lid is also filled with a beverage such as tea, a fruit infusion or lemon/lime water that I put into my bag & carry with me wherever I am going.

3) I have two small plastic containers ~ One that hold nuts & seeds, such as macadamia nuts, pistachio nuts, pumpkin seeds, sunflower seeds, soaked almonds, etc. In the second small container I take a healthy, raw, organic trail mix such as *Activated Sprouted Trail Mix* or *Go Take a Hike*. If I am short on time, I may simplify with one of my favorite combos which is macadamia nuts & golden berries. That way, I have something sweet & salty in one small container.

4) In one green medium size container, I take sliced organic fresh fruit such as apples, oranges, pears, kiwi, pineapple, longans, whatever is in season. It usually takes less than 5 minutes to wash, slice & pack them. Then I place that green plastic container inside the small size thermal bag with blue ice.

5) If I am going to be out for a longer time, I fill a second green medium size container with raw fresh sliced veggies such as carrots, celery, red pepper, green pepper, jicama, etc. I also include my favorite olives that are super yum! They are ~ Sunfood Organic Pitted Peruvian Black Botija Olives, Divina Organic Pitted Green Olives & Divina Organic Kalamata Olives.

6) In the 3rd small container, I put a yummy cashew/ macadamia nut dip or homemade hummus in which to dip the sliced veggies.
(Recipe for the nut dip is on page 270 & the recipe for hummus is on page 277.)

So, whenever I leave the house, I have something yin & yang, sweet & savory with me. This way I am never in a situation that I let my blood sugar level drop. This supports me to maintain steady, balanced, energy to feel my best & have my best to give.

This may all seem like a big deal to you at first, but I assure you that once you get these simple systems in place, it is so quick, easy & worthwhile! Then you are never tempted to reach for something that would not be beneficial for your mind, body & Spirit!

When we take the time to plan, pack & be prepared, it is such a small price to pay for radiant wellbeing!

Health truly is our greatest wealth because without it, it is very difficult to achieve our best, whether it be spiritual or material.

There are two kinds of discomfort, one comes from discipline, which I prefer to think of as devotion, and the other comes from dealing with the fallout from not being disciplined/devoted.

I have come to the ***clear*** realization that it is sooooo much easier to deal with the discomfort of discipline than it is to deal with the consequences of not being disciplined, such as being disorganized, unprepared, self-recriminating or experiencing a lower level of health, self-esteem & wellbeing on every level.

I love this quote by Jim Rohn. *"We must all suffer from one of two pains: the pain of discipline or the pain of regret. The difference is discipline weighs ounces while regret weighs tons."*

"First you form your habits, then they form you," so why not choose & implement the habits that put you on an upward spiral of health & wellbeing!

The goal of all goals is to feel good so set yourself up to feel your best. Then you have your best to give & everyone wins!

Getting Set Up

"Preparing food is love made visible."

Because health truly is our greatest wealth, I highly recommend investing in a few kitchen appliances that make a world of difference in healthy food preparation. These are items that you can use day in & day out. Having them really sets you up to succeed because they make it so easy, practical & time efficient to prepare healthy food.

Although I lean toward eating mainly raw food, there are times, especially on colder or rainier days when warm food feels more grounding & comforting.

Here is my support team in the kitchen ~

* Vitamix ~ Ideal for smoothies, dressings, dips, "blisscream" & making fresh flour.

* Food Processor ~ Ideal for peanut butter, cilantro coconut chutney, macadamia nut ricotta, bliss balls, etc.

* Rice Cooker ~ Ideal for cooking any grains.

* Instant Pot ~ Ideal for cooking beans & soups.

* Air Fryer ~ Ideal for no-oil French fries, crispy garbanzo bean snack & oil-free cookies.

* Toaster Oven ~ Ideal for baked patties such as falafel, without heating up the whole house & wasting energy heating up a big oven.

* Coffee/seed grinder ~ Ideal for making instant fresh flour, grinding seeds & spices.

* Eco-friendly, stick-free griddle ~ Ideal for oil-free flat breads & pancakes.

If you eat mainly raw, you might want to consider investing in a juicer & a dehydrator.

What I love about the rice cooker, Instant Pot, air fryer & toaster oven is that you don't have to babysit them. You set them up to go & they turn themselves off. That way, once you set them up, you can go about your day & when you return, voila, like magic, your food is ready!

I use ceramic knives in 3 sizes that make a world of difference in food preparation! Ceramic knives have also been proven to stay sharp for up to 10 times longer than metal knives.

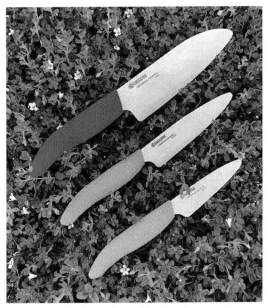

Photo by Julie Stuehser

There are countless delicious & nutritious vegan recipes. Below are a few of my favorite go-to recipes to get started. I have also included a resource section at the end of this book to explore an abundance of other great recipes.

All of my recipes use straight-from-the-source, non-processed or minimally processed, organic, non-GMO ingredients, whenever possible.

In addition to using fresh, whole organic ingredients, the way in which you prepare the food and the energy that you infuse it with is also vitally important. As Tesla said, *"Everything is energy, frequency & vibration."*

This is why I begin by cleaning my food preparation surfaces with my handy dandy spray bottle of hydrogen peroxide & then I wash my hands thoroughly with a vegan, organic non-toxic soap such as *Dr. Bronner's* soap or *100% Pure* before beginning.

Then, whenever possible, I light a candle or two as I set my intention to proceed as meditation in action & devotion in motion. While preparing food, I often listen to uplifting devotional music & inspiring talks on my laptop computer.

I infuse the food that I am preparing with love, mantras & immense gratitude for our abundance of fresh organic food, purified water & all of our favorable conditions!

I offer the food to the Divine before ingesting it with a prayer of gratitude. I pray that the prana (life-force energy) from this food fuel me to be the best instrument of Divine Benevolence that I can be.

You can use or create any sacred rituals and prayers that resonate with you.

Enjoy in good health & bon appetit!

Angel's Basic Template for a Balanced Healthy Diet

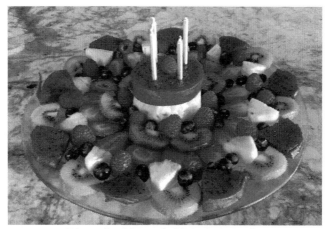

Photo by Meenakshi Angel Honig

Many people are convinced that a plant-based diet is the healthiest, most compassionate & sustainable choice but they just don't know how to go about making the transition.

So here is my basic template for a balanced, healthy, unprocessed, or minimally processed diet. It consists of organic fruit, vegetables, sea vegetables, mushrooms, whole grains, beans & legumes, nuts, seeds, sprouts, fresh herbs & freshly ground whole spices.

There are many great health benefits for starting off your day with some purified water with fresh squeezed lemon in it.

According to *Healthline*, lemons contain a high amount of vitamin C, soluble fiber & plant compounds. As a rich source of vitamin C, lemon juice protects the body from immune system deficiencies. Drinking lemon juice with warm water every morning helps in maintaining the pH balance of your body temple & acts as a detoxifying agent. Lemon water may also aid in weight loss, reducing your risk of heart disease, anemia, kidney stones, digestive issues & cancer.

Lemon juice can affect the enamel on your teeth so I recommend drinking it with a reusable straw to bypass the teeth. It is also a good practice to rinse your mouth with purified water after drinking lemon water to remove any residual acidity.

I put my purified water in mason jars & place them outside on my lanai overnight, so that the water gets a solar & lunar charge. It also gets charged with a sound bath from the melodious choir of the very happy neighborhood birds who frequent here & sing enthusiastically!

Given that *"everything is energy, frequency & vibration,"* I also charge the water I drink with gratitude. I ask that it purify me, as well as water the fruition of my Angel missions for the highest good of all.

A few good choices for the morning, depending on the unique circumstances of each day, are celery juice, smoothies, a fresh fruit salad sprinkled with sprouted trail mix or sliced apples dipped in homemade peanut/macadamia nut butter.
(Recipe for peanut/macadamia nut butter is on page 284.)

I, personally, like to do intermittent fasting, (not that I recommend it for everyone), so on most mornings, I just have lemon water & organic green tea.

Lunch & dinner center around a robust, colorful salad or a hearty Buddha bowl.

A Buddha bowl may mean different things to different people. For me, the anatomy of an ideal Buddha bowl is an artistic, delicious & nutritious layering of any grain, any legume, rainbow salad & homemade sauerkraut, drizzled with creamy dressing.

Recipes for ~

★ Rainbow salads on page 246

★ Sauerkraut on page 287

★ Creamy Dressing on page 270

★ Buddha bowls on page 250

A Divine Romance

Grains & beans make an ideal pair because together they contain all nine essential amino acids that form a complete source of protein. Most traditional cuisines have been in love with this combination in different forms for over 10,000 years, such as Mexican rice & beans, Indian rice & dhal, Asian rice & tofu, Mideastern hummus & pita bread, just to name a few.

When selecting your grains & legumes, let's avoid getting stuck in the same old, same old. Play with a wide variety of grains such as ~

Grains

★ Rice ~ There are so many different varieties to choose from such as brown, basmati, wild, sprouted, biodynamic, arborio, forbidden rice, jasmine & japonic rice

★ Millet   ★ Buckwheat
★ Quinoa   ★ Bulgar
★ Farro   ★ Oats
★ Kamut   ★ Spelt
★ Amaranth   ★ Barley

Beans & Legumes

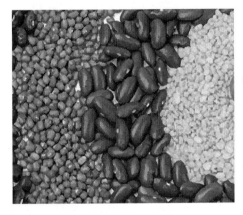 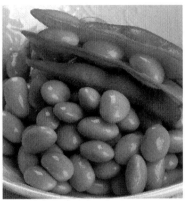

- Aduki Beans
  (Also known as Azuki Beans)
- Bean Sprouts
- Black Beans
- Black-Eyed Peas
- Calypso (Yin Yang) Beans
- Cannellini Beans
- Edamame
- Fava Beans
- Garbanzo Beans
- Green Beans
- Lima Beans
- Lentils, brown, green, yellow & red
- Mung Beans
- Navy Beans
- Northern Beans
- Pea Pods & Green Peas
- Pinto Beans
- Red Beans
- Soy Beans, black & red
- Wax Beans
- Kidney Beans
- White Beans

I suggest having two plastic bins in your fridge, one with an assortment of grains & the other with a variety of beans & legumes.

When I am ready to prepare the grain & legume du jour, I bring the two bins out onto the kitchen counter & ask my *body*, (not my mind), to tune into which grain & legume has the nutrients that would be best for that particular day. Notice what you gravitate to when you ask your *body* that question.

Then I rinse & soak the desired amount of each. It is ideal to soak the beans & grains overnight or for 8 hours, however a shorter time is still beneficial. As Voltaire said, *"Don't let perfection be the enemy of good."*

I put the grain in the rice cooker & the beans in the instant pot. I just set them up, press 'play' & go about my day! Then, when I return, voila, they are ready to enjoy!

Sea Vegetables

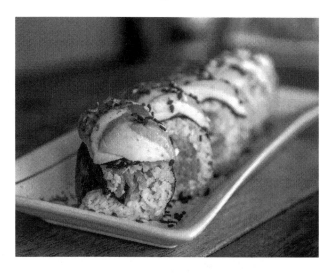

Sea veggies are deliciously rich in fiber & are one of the most alkalizing foods on the planet. They are a great source of vitamins & trace minerals such as iron, magnesium, calcium & potassium. Sea vegetables are also full of antioxidant compounds that help to remove heavy metals & toxic pollutants from our body temples.

Here are a few to add to salads, soups, grains & bean dishes. They also come in flakes, in convenient shakers, that you can sprinkle on your food, as desired.

- ★ Nori
- ★ Kelp
- ★ Kombu
- ★ Wakame
- ★ Dulse
- ★ Laver
- ★ Hijiki
- ★ Arame

Nuts & Seeds

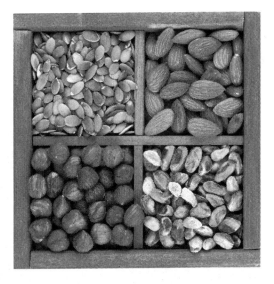

Nuts & seeds are great sources of protein, healthy fats, fiber, vitamins, minerals & are powerhouses for antioxidants.

Many people avoid eating nuts because they think that they are high in fat & calories, however research shows that eating nuts may actually help to regulate weight because their fats are not fully absorbed. Despite being high in fat, nuts have a number of impressive health and weight loss benefits.

Nuts are one of the healthiest snacks you can eat, because they contain a wide range of essential nutrients. These health benefits are attributed to nuts that have been minimally processed and have no added ingredients. Many processed nut products, such as peanut butter, often contain high amounts of salt, added oil & sugar. So, it's best to buy nuts as close to their natural state as possible. I am astounded by how quick & easy it is to make your own fresh delicious nut butters at home!
(See page 284 for the recipe.)

Here are some of the health benefits of eating nuts from *Healthline* ~

1) **Nuts are highly nutritious** ~ One ounce (28 grams) of mixed nuts contains ~

★ Calories: 173

★ Protein: 5 grams

★ Fat: 16 grams, including 9 grams of monounsaturated fat

★ Carbs: 6 grams

★ Fiber: 3 grams

★ Vitamin E: 12% of the RDI

★ Magnesium: 16% of the RDI

★ Phosphorus: 13% of the RDI

★ Copper: 23% of the RDI

★ Manganese: 26% of the RDI

★ Selenium: 56% of the RDI

2) **Nuts are loaded with Antioxidants** ~ Nuts contain antioxidants known as polyphenols, which may protect your cells from damage caused by free radicals.

3) **May Aid Weight Loss** ~ Nuts have been shown to promote weight loss rather than contribute to weight gain. Several studies indicate that your body doesn't absorb all of the calories in nuts.

4) **May Lower Cholesterol & Triglycerides** ~ Research indicates that nuts may help lower "bad" LDL cholesterol & triglycerides while boosting levels of "good" HDL cholesterol.

5) **Beneficial for Type 2 Diabetes & Metabolic Syndrome** ~ Several studies have shown that blood sugar, blood pressure & other health markers improve when people with type 2 diabetes & metabolic syndrome include nuts in their diet.

6) **May Reduce Inflammation** ~ Research suggests that nuts may reduce inflammation, especially in people with diabetes, kidney disease & other serious health conditions.

7) **High in Beneficial Fiber** ~ Many nuts are high in fiber, which can help keep you full, decrease calorie absorption & improve gut health.

8) **May Reduce Your Risk of Heart Attack & Stroke** ~ Nuts may significantly lower your risk of heart attack & stroke. Eating nuts increases "bad" LDL particle size, raises "good" HDL cholesterol, improves artery function & has various other benefits. (Many recent studies have looked into the importance of LDL particle size. Studies show that people whose LDL particles are predominantly small & dense, have a threefold greater risk of coronary heart disease. Furthermore, the large and fluffy type of LDL may be protective.)

Here are some great nuts to include in your everyday food choices ~

- ★ Almonds
- ★ Pistachio
- ★ Walnuts
- ★ Cashews
- ★ Peanuts
- ★ Macadamia
- ★ Brazil Nuts
- ★ Hazel Nuts
- ★ Pine Nuts
- ★ Pecans

(Although peanuts are technically legumes, they are commonly referred to as nuts due to their similar nutrition profile & characteristics.)

Seeds

Hemp Seeds ~ A great source of protein, rich in healthy essential fatty acids, high in vitamin E, phosphorus, potassium, sodium, magnesium, sulfur, calcium, iron & zinc.

Flax Seeds ~ Are high in omega-3 fats, rich in high quality protein, antioxidants & fiber.

Chia Seeds ~ Deliver a massive amount of nutrients with very few calories & are loaded with high quality protein, omega-3 fatty acids & fiber.

Pumpkin Seeds ~ Are high in protein, antioxidants, magnesium & fiber.

Sunflower Seeds ~ Are rich in the B complex vitamins & are a good source of phosphorus, magnesium, iron, calcium, potassium, protein & vitamin E.

Sesame Seeds ~ Are a great source of healthy fats, protein, B vitamins, minerals, fiber & antioxidants.

Nuts & Seeds are easy to incorporate into your everyday diet

Nuts & seeds are a great high protein snack. They are easy to pack in your lunch, keep in your purse or bag, have in your car or at your desk so that they are readily available whenever you need a quick, healthy snack to keep your blood sugar level even.

Blood sugar, or glucose, is the main sugar found in your blood. It comes from the food you eat & is your body's main source of energy. Your blood carries glucose to all of your body's cells to use for energy. Have you ever noticed how some people get grouchy, fatigued or brain fog when their blood sugar level drops? A steady even blood sugar level makes for a steady mind, focused concentration & balanced moods.

You can also add nuts & seeds to ~

- ★ Smoothies
- ★ Dressings
- ★ Trail mixes
- ★ Fruit salads
- ★ Oatmeal
- ★ Stir-fries
- ★ Veggie salads
- ★ Nut milks
- ★ Nut butters
- ★ Crackers
- ★ Baked goods
- ★ Falafel
- ★ Nut burgers
- ★ Buddha bowls

Make Room for Mushrooms

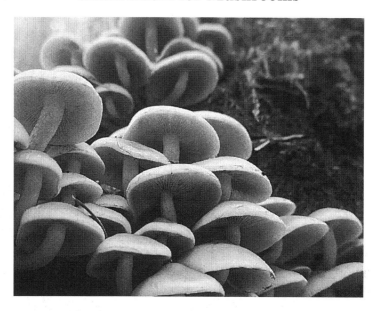

Although mushrooms are classified as vegetables, technically they are not plants but part of the kingdom called fungi.

According to Dr. Joel Fuhrman, *"Mushrooms seem to be almost magical in promoting health benefits. From fighting respiratory infections to cancer, this assortment of small fungi are gigantic warriors."*

Unlike most other vegetables, mushrooms contain two important B vitamins; niacin & riboflavin. The shiitake is a particularly healthful mushroom, as it contains lentinan, which may help fight cancer & bolster the immune system.

Here a few of the amazing benefits from *Food.ndtv.com* for including mushrooms in your daily diet.

★ **Checks Cholesterol Levels** ~ Mushrooms are full of lean proteins and have negligible fat or cholesterol.

★ **Maintains Bone Health** ~ Mushrooms contain abundant calcium which is an essential nutrient to maintain strong bones.

★ **Boosts the Immune System** ~ Out of the many antioxidants present in mushrooms, ergothioneine is an antioxidant that is effective in protecting your body from free radicals.

★ **Good for Diabetics** ~ According to Dr. Simran Saini, *"Mushrooms are a great source of chromium which helps maintain blood sugar levels further keeping a check on insulin & thus it is a super food for diabetics."*

★ **Helps in Weight Loss** ~ Mushrooms contain a lot of fiber which contributes to improving digestion & keeps the metabolism in check. Mushrooms do not contain any fat or carbohydrates so they are ideal to add to any weight loss plan.

* **Breast Cancer Prevention** ~ According to Dr. Fuhrman, one notable study found frequent consumption of mushrooms (10g, or approximately one button mushroom per day) has been linked to a 64% decrease in the risk of breast cancer! Mushrooms are thought to protect against breast cancer particularly because they inhibit an enzyme called aromatase, which produces estrogen. Several varieties of mushrooms, especially the commonly eaten white button & portobello mushrooms, have strong anti-aromatase activity.

* **Protects the brain from oxidative stress** ~ According to Dr. Fuhrman, mushrooms are the richest dietary source of the specialized antioxidant ergothioneine; all mushrooms contain some ergothioneine, but oyster mushrooms contain the most. Studies on dietary factors & cognitive health in older adults, particularly in Asia, have found that greater mushroom consumption or ergothioneine levels in the blood were associated with better brain health.

Enjoy a variety of mushrooms such as ~

* White Button
* Crimini
* Portabello
* Shiitake
* Maitake
* Oyster
* Enoki

* Reishi
* Porcini
* Morel
* Beech
* Chanterelle
* Black Trumpet
* King Trumpet

Some studies indicate that raw mushrooms, even common button mushrooms, contain small traces of carcinogenic compounds such as hydrazine & a naturally occurring formaldehyde. Both chemicals are heat-sensitive & are destroyed by cooking.

Also, some of the anti-cancer effects of eating mushrooms are more absorbed when eating cooked mushrooms because cooking breaks down the cell walls of the mushrooms making the nutrients more bioavailable.

Mushrooms can be steamed, sautéed, baked, broiled, grilled & dried.

Mushrooms have a uniquely savory umami flavor & are especially tasty in lentil barley soup, gravies & stir-fries. (I stir-fry with water rather than oil.)

Due to their meat-like texture, mushrooms can serve as a good substitute for those transitioning to a vegan diet.

No Doubt, It's a Miracle to Sprout!

There are countless benefits for growing & incorporating sprouts into your diet.

A few of the health benefits include ~

★ Aids in digestion

★ Improves blood circulation

★ Helps lose weight

* Builds immune system

* Improves eye sight

* Regulates cholesterol level

* Heart friendly ~ According to *organicmicrogreens.uk* sprouts have omega-3 fatty acids which help in boosting good cholesterol (HDL) levels & reduce the amount of harmful cholesterol in your blood vessels & arteries.

* Omega-3 fatty acids have anti-inflammatory properties that help in reducing the excessive stress on your cardiovascular system.

* The presence of potassium helps reduce blood pressure levels, further reducing the risk of any cardiovascular problem.

* Reduces acidity ~ Many illnesses, including cancer, are associated with excess acidity in the body.

* Sprouts are alkalizing to the body. They help regulate and maintain the pH levels of your body by reducing the level of acids.

* Rejuvenates hair & skin

* Helps to reduce premature aging

A Miraculous Garden in a Jar in your own Kitchen!

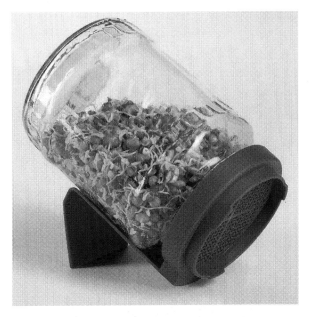

"In the garden of dreams, there are many great seeds of possibilities waiting to sprout - looking for your attention - the water & the light." - Amit Ray

There are a wide variety of amazing sprouts that you can grow in your own kitchen! Edible sprouts are superfoods that can be grown all year round.

Sprouts are excellent sources of protein, antioxidants, essential amino acids, vitamins & minerals. Sprouts can grow from the seeds of vegetables, grains, legumes, buckwheat & beans. Alfalfa sprouts are one of the most popular sprout varieties known around the world.

A few types of Sprouts are ~

- Alfalfa
- Radish
- Mung Bean
- Broccoli
- Clover
- Beet
- Fenugreek

- Quinoi
- Barley
- Soy Beans
- Buckwheat
- Black beans
- Sunflower
- Peas

- Mustard
- Lentil
- Garbanzo
- Chives
- Cabbage
- Adzuki
- Onion Sprouts

Some wonderful benefits of eating sprouts from the *Sproutman.com*

- Home sprouting is significantly cheaper than buying organic produce.

- Sprouts are always in season.

- It takes just a few minutes of attention per day.

- No soil, no pesticides, no bugs.

- No special light or temperature is required.

- Lettuce in your local supermarket can actually be a week to a month old by the time you buy it. Why eat a dead salad when you can nourish yourself with an organic, living one?

★ Since sprouts of any variety are technically still living when you eat them, there is no loss of nutrients post-harvest, unlike their full-grown counterparts that have been chopped from their roots.

★ Sprouts are the most sustainable form of produce you can get year-round.

★ They have a much smaller carbon footprint than refrigerated market veggies, since they take up much less space in transport, require no soil, fertilizer or pesticides & don't need refrigeration to get from the garden to your plate.

★ When you support the sprouting seed industry, you are encouraging farmers to grow & harvest organic sprouting seeds rather than conventional or bioengineered seeds. It is simple supply & demand and has a powerful impact on environmental outcomes.

★ One pound of sprouts only requires 9 inches of space! You can even grow them in a bag & hang them so that they don't take up precious kitchen real estate.

★ Whether you live in a tiny studio apartment, a massive multi-bedroom estate with acres of gardens or are getting prepped for a nomadic year of van life, you can easily sprout your beans & greens right in your kitchen, no matter the size.

★ Instead of farm-to-table, how about kitchen to table?

Creative ideas for incorporating more sprouts into your diet

★ Sprouts make a nutritious salad base.

★ Mix varieties like daikon radish, broccoli blend & a salad mix for a flavorful bed of greens.

★ Blend into green smoothies.

★ Sprout garbanzo beans for a delicious sprouted hummus.

★ Bake into breads & muffins, or even make sprouted wheat pizza!

★ Sauté sprouted beans to make nutrient-rich stir-fries & taco fillings. (I stir-fry in water or veggie broth rather than oil.)

★ Season, mix & dehydrate sprouts to make tasty sprouted crackers!

★ For more ideas, check out some of the Sproutman's classic recipes in *Sproutman's Kitchen Garden Cookbook* & *Sprouts: The Miracle Food*.

Broccoli Sprouts

"Just Do it!" - Nike's iconic motto

Broccoli sprouts have astounding health benefits & they are so simple to sprout!

A while back my sister's husband, Steve, sent me a package of broccoli seeds to sprout. He shared his enthusiasm about the amazing health benefits so I gave it a try. Broccoli seeds are really easy to sprout & they have a kind of radish-like taste that adds a blast of flavor & nutrition to your salads.

When I rinse the sprouts twice a day, I infuse them with love, gratitude & mantras. It is a wonderful feeling to watch them grow, to be connected with the process & to participate in the miracle of life!

Here are a few of the health benefits of broccoli sprouts to inspire you to, *"Just do it!"* You will be glad you did.

Some Health Benefits of Broccoli Sprouts

★ Organic broccoli sprouts are one of the most popular varieties of sprouts & have more documented anti-cancer efficacy than any other sprout.

★ This includes research on their anti-tumor properties, effective against a wide range of cancers, such as prostate, breast, bladder, stomach & skin cancer.

★ For those who consume these cruciferous sprouts, the high glucosinolate content in broccoli converts upon digestion to sulforaphane, which induces "phase 2 enzymes" that significantly slow the production of human cancer cells.

According to *ProHealth.com*, ingesting broccoli sprouts ~

★ Reduces autism symptoms

★ Promotes the healing of TBI (Traumatic Brain Injury)

★ Inhibits neurodegenerative disease

★ Alleviates depression & anxiety

★ Promotes detoxification

★ Has antibacterial effects

★ Contains sulforaphane which has antimicrobial effects against a wide range of human pathogens

★ Alleviates autoimmunity

★ Boosts the immune system

★ Alleviates asthma & lung inflammation

★ Protects skin from UV damage

★ Promotes prevention & treatment of cancer

★ Improves heart health

★ Combats obesity

★ Promotes bone health

★ It takes just a few days from seed to salad!

★ Checking out the *sproutman.com* website is a good way to get started.

★ No doubt, it is a miracle to sprout!

Growing Broccoli Sprouts in 5 Easy Steps

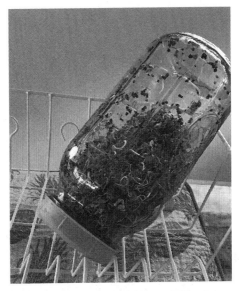

Photo by Meenakshi Angel Honig

1) Add two tablespoons of broccoli seeds, to a wide-mouthed glass jar. Cover with a few inches of purified water & cap with the sprouting lid. Store in a warm, dark place overnight. (Or, you can use a sprout bag.)

2) 8 hours later, drain off the water & rinse with fresh water. Drain the fresh water.

3) Place the sprouting jar upside down at a 45-degree angle on a sprouting jar stand or in your dish rack. Place in the sunlight.

4) Rinse & drain the sprouts twice a day for approximately 4 - 5 days or until the sprouts are dark green.

5) Once the sprouts are dark green, they are ready to eat! They are great to add to salads & wraps. You can store the sprouts in a mason jar with a standard lid in the fridge.

Using Whole Spices & Fresh Herbs

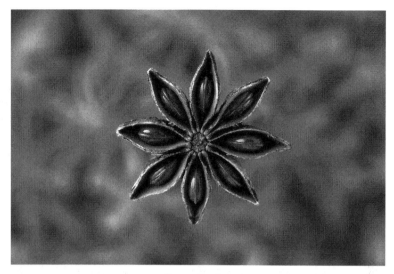

Star Anise

Spices & herbs have been used for centuries for both culinary & medicinal purposes. They are a great way to add flavor, aroma & color to our food & beverages without adding extra fat, sugar or salt. They also provide powerful antioxidants & deliver an astounding array of health benefits!

I use whole spices & fresh herbs in place of ground ones because as I mentioned earlier, unprocessed food is more hygienic in that it is not inadvertently ground up with insect fragments & other disgusting debris. Fresh whole spices & herbs are also much more fragrant & potent than the ground version. Of course, you can also use the processed ground spices & herbs in these recipes, if you prefer.

- ★ **Cardamon** ~ Take the cardamon seeds out of the pods. The seeds can be used whole or you can grind freshly in a coffee/spice grinder.

- ★ **Nutmeg** ~ Take a whole nutmeg & hold your grater at about a 45 degree angle. Grate & be 'grateful' when you breathe in that 'grate' Divine fragrance! The best kind of grater to use is a microplane grater because it has sharper edges than a standard grater. Nutmeg has many health benefits in small amounts, however as little as 2 teaspoons or 5 grams can cause some symptoms of toxicity, so use it sparingly.

- ★ **Cinnamon** ~ Place your cinnamon sticks into a manual or automatic coffee/spice grinder. If the sticks are too long, break them into smaller pieces so the lid of the grinder can close securely. Start the grinder & run until the cinnamon has been completely pulverized.

- ★ **Cloves** ~ Can be used whole or grind freshly in a coffee/spice grinder. Use them sparingly because they tend to overpower more delicate spices.

- ★ **Star Anise** ~ The star anise pod is shaped like a star & has an average of eight points. Each point contains a single seed. Both the seeds & the pod can be used whole or ground freshly in a coffee/spice grinder for a sweet licorice-peppery flavor.

- ★ **Coriander Seeds** ~ Use whole or grind freshly in a coffee/spice grinder.

- ★ **Cumin Seed** ~ Use whole or grind freshly in a coffee/spice grinder.

- ★ **Fenugreek Seeds** ~ Use whole or grind freshly in a coffee/spice grinder.

- ★ **Black Mustard Seed**s ~ Dry roast in non-stick pan until they pop.

- ★ **Saffron** ~ Its subtle taste & aroma pairs well with savory dishes such as risottos, dhal & rice dishes. The best way to draw out saffron's unique flavor is to soak the threads in hot (not boiling) water.

- ★ **Tamarind** ~ Remove the reddish, brown colored paste from the seeds in the pod. Add the paste to savory recipes for a sweet & sour, rich base note flavor. I like to use it in recipes that call for soy sauce & vegan Worcestershire sauce because when you take the paste from the pod, it is straight-from-the-source & unprocessed.

- ★ **Pink & Black Himalayan Salt Crystals** ~ This table & cooking salt is readily available & can be easily purchased in a convenient refillable mill with a ceramic grinder.

- ★ **Pepper** ~ Black, green or white varieties are best freshly ground from the peppercorns. They are readily available, packaged in convenient refillable mills which makes it so quick & easy to grind freshly each time.

Using Fresh Herbs

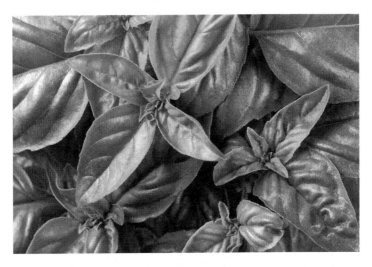

In addition to being more hygienic & potent, fresh herbs bring your recipes to life, making them pop with fresh flavor, aroma, color & prana, (life-force energy)!

Here are some delectable fresh herbs that you can grow in your own kitchen, on your deck or purchase at farmers markets, health food stores & at local grocery stores.

- ★ Basil
- ★ Parsley
- ★ Cilantro
- ★ Dill
- ★ Thyme
- ★ Oregano
- ★ Chives
- ★ Fennel
- ★ Sage
- ★ Tarragon
- ★ Mint
- ★ Rosemary

Honoring the Season & the Life-force

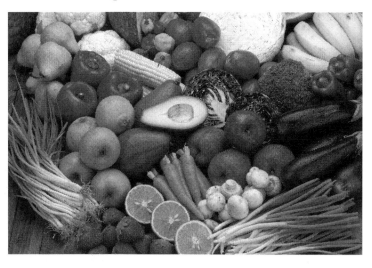

As I mentioned earlier this is not a diet; it is a mindset & a lifestyle.

I am so grateful that I can place a weekly produce order for fresh fruits & veggies that are in season, with a local farm-to-table organic farmer, who delivers every week. It is worth checking to see what organic produce options are available in your area. I highly encourage going to your local Farmer's markets whenever possible &, of course, growing your own produce if you can. Even if you are not in a position to have a full-blown garden, just having a few pots of fresh herbs growing on your porch can bring your salads to life!

Because I eat a *straight-from-the-source, unprocessed or minimally processed* vegan diet, my daily meals are largely dictated by honoring the life-force of the produce that I have on hand. So, when I open the fridge, I assess what needs to be used first, in order to honor its life-force & then I center my menu around that.

It is also beneficial to honor the life-force in everything, to the best of our ability, to decrease waste. For example, I had a wonderful assistant who was helping me move. At the completion of our successful mission, she commented that she had learned so much by working side-by-side with me for the previous few days. I was curious as to what, in particular, she had picked up & so I asked her to give me an example of one thing that she learned. She said that she learned to honor the life-force in a paper towel.

Although I prefer to use washable towels whenever possible, there are those occasions when a paper towel is called for. Whenever I use a paper towel, I don't like to discard it until I have fully honored its life-force. So, if it was just used to dry hands, I like to use it to run along the baseboards in the house, picking up any dust, before discarding it. In this way, I honor its life-force, instead of tossing it out before it is fully used.

The mindful application of honoring the life-force can spill over into other areas of your life, infusing an attitude of reverence toward all life.

Angel's Favorite Go-To Meals

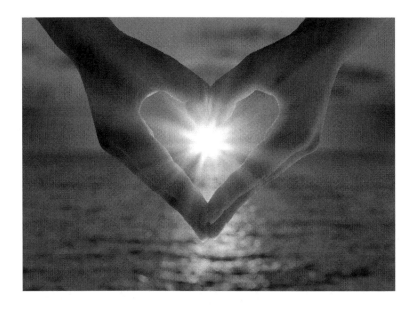

"The main ingredient is Love"

Here are a few of my favorite go-to meals to get started, followed by my recipes.

Breakfast Options
- ★ Super Green Smoothie
- ★ Super Violet Flame Smoothie
- ★ Mango Lassi Smoothie
- ★ Oatmeal with Superfoods
- ★ Vanilla Chia Pudding

Lunch Options

- ★ Vibrant Rainbow Salads
- ★ Fulfilling Buddha Bowls
- ★ Ziggy's Zalad
- ★ Zoodles with Avocado Pesto Sauce
- ★ Romaine Rolls & Love Boats
- ★ Super Yum Sandwich, Taco, Tostada, Wrap, Burrito or 'Mini Pizza'

Dinner Options

- ★ Creamy Vibrant Green Comfort Soup
- ★ Fabulous Falafel on Savory Flatbread
- ★ Air French Fries with Rainbow Salad
- ★ Vegetable Dhal with Basmati Rice
- ★ A Medley of Steamed Veggies drizzled with Peanut Macadamia Nut Sauce
- ★ Angel Hair "Pasta" with Pesto Sauce

Flatbreads

- ★ Chapati Flatbread
- ★ Lentil Flatbread
- ★ Potato Pancakes

Dressings, Dips, 'Cheezes', Sauces, Gravy, Nut Butters, Chutney & Sauerkraut

- ★ Creamy Cashew Dressing & Dip
- ★ Ricotta Macadamia Nut 'Cheeze'
- ★ Lemon Tahini Dressing & Dipping Sauce
- ★ Green Goddess Avocado Dressing
- ★ Almond Lime Dressing
- ★ Hummus
- ★ Presto Pesto
- ★ Guacamole
- ★ Savory Gravy
- ★ Cilantro Coconut Chutney
- ★ Nut Butters
- ★ Peanut Macadamia Nut Sauce
- ★ Cashew Cream
- ★ Sauerkraut

Delectable Desserts

- ★ Frozen Cherries, Blueberries & Strawberries
- ★ Heavenly Fruit Salad
- ★ Dreamboat Dates
- ★ Ginger Joy Balls
- ★ Raw Cacao Bliss Balls
- ★ Berry "Blisscream" (Vegan ice cream)

Snacks

- ★ Macadamia Nuts with Golden Berries
- ★ Pistachio Nuts
- ★ Raw Trailmix with Golden Berries
- ★ Steamed Edamame
- ★ Soaked Almonds & Raisins
- ★ Sliced Fresh Fruit
- ★ Sliced Raw Veggies Dipped in Hummus
- ★ Celery & Apples Dipped in Peanut/Macadamia nut Butter
- ★ Black & Green Olives
- ★ Crispy Roasted Garbanzo Beans
- ★ Presto Pesto Popcorn
- ★ Avocado "Toast"

Refreshing Beverages

- ★ Ginger Turmeric Tea
- ★ Lemongrass Mint Tea
- ★ Green Tea with a Squeeze of Lemon or Lime
- ★ Rejuvenating Rejuvelac
- ★ Fruit Infusions
- ★ Homemade Almond Milk
- ★ Golden Turmeric Almond Milk
- ★ Homemade Chai Tea with Almond Date Milk
- ★ Goddess Lemon-'aid'
- ★ Angel's Cinnamon Water

Angel's Recipes

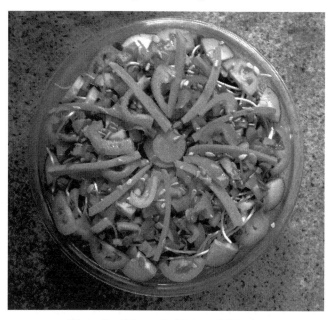

Photo by Meenakshi Angel Honig

Here are a few of my favorite recipes to get started. Because I prepare my food by feel rather than by measuring it, my dear friends, Julie Stuehser & Rebecca French helped me to come up with some approximate measurements. These estimates sorely lack surgical precision. So, I invite you to be playful & creative in the kitchen & make the recipes to the proportions that are most appealing to you. You really can't get it wrong. For example, if you add an extra mango here or another banana there in your smoothies, they are still going to be awesome! Each one is unique, just like you!

What makes my recipes unique is that all of these recipes use straight-from-the-source, unprocessed, or minimally processed, ingredients. This means there are no commercially ground spices or flour, no added oil or sugar & no other processed foods because these items, as I mentioned earlier, inadvertently include insect fragments & other disgusting debris. Please refer to the FDA Food Defect Levels Handbook that I referenced on page 187 to see for yourself.

I use organic, non-GMO ingredients whenever possible. By embracing food the way that nature brings it, without all the artificial additives, preservatives, toxins & debris, we spiral ourselves up to a higher frequency of wellbeing!

I'd like to share something with you that I find amusing. One of the most challenging parts for me in putting this recipe section together was coming up with the measurements because as I mentioned, I have always done food preparation by feel & not by measuring.

So, I bought myself a set of shiny stainless steel measuring cups & spoons. I then embarked on preparing my recipes & reverse engineering to figure out the measurements. This was not an easy task because I always improvise with whatever fresh ingredients I have on hand & so each batch is different.

In any case, by Divine Grace, diligent effort & a little help from my friends, I was able to come up with some approximate measurements.

Today, I wanted to make some fresh peanut butter. So, rather than play the guessing game, I went to my own recipe book & followed the recipe for peanut macadamia nut butter & it came out perfectly! So, now I am consulting my own recipe book to make my own recipes! This just strikes me as funny! :):)

Isn't it great when the right brain & left brain work & play together!

Recipes for Breakfast Options

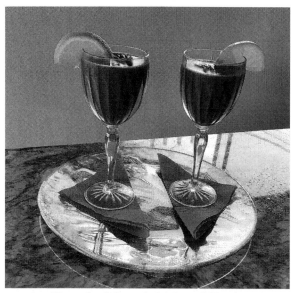

Photo by Meenakshi Angel Honig

Super Green Smoothie

Green smoothies are a fresh, delicious, energizing way to launch your day!

- ★ Oranges, peeled ~ 3
- ★ Spinach or kale, or a combination thereof ~ a large handful
- ★ Cilantro & Basil ~ to taste
- ★ Four Super Foods: flax seeds, chia seeds, hemp seeds & raw cacao nibs (not cacao powder) ~ 1 teaspoon each
- ★ Fresh vanilla bean, chopped ~ 2 inches
- ★ Frozen bananas ~ 3
- ★ Ice ~ 1 - 2 cups
- ★ Purified water ~ as needed for desired consistency to blend & pour smoothly
- ★ Mantras, Love & Gratitude ~ copious amounts!

1) Wash & blend the ingredients. Enjoy!

Variation ~

★ Experiment with different fruits, greens, nuts & seeds to discover your favorite go-to smoothie.

Tips ~

1) Smoothies blend best when you place the juiciest fruits, such as oranges, at the bottom closest to the blades.

2) I find that smoothies blend more smoothly when I blend in stages. For example, blend all the ingredients above except the frozen bananas & ice to get a liquid mass. Then add the frozen bananas & ice to that mixture ~ a cool & smooth move! :)

Super Violet Flame Smoothie

This smoothie is a gorgeous life-giving violet color!

★ Oranges, peeled ~ 3

★ Frozen strawberries, blueberries & pitted cherries ~ totaling 2 cups

★ Cilantro ~ to taste

★ Basil ~ to taste

★ Four Super Foods: flax seeds, chia seeds, hemp seeds & raw cacao nibs (not cacao powder) ~ 1 teaspoon each

★ Fresh vanilla bean chopped ~ 2 inches

★ Frozen bananas ~ 3

★ Ice ~ 1 - 2 cups

★ Purified Water ~ as needed for desired consistency to blend & pour smoothly.

1) Wash, blend & enjoy!

Tips ~

1) Smoothies blend best when you place the juiciest fruits, such as oranges at the bottom, closest to the blades.

2) I find that blending in stages works more smoothly. For example, I blend the oranges, bananas, cilantro, basil, super foods & vanilla to get a liquid mass. Then I add the frozen berries & ice to that mixture. This makes it easier to blend overall.

Mango Lassi Smoothie ~ Ambrosia Nectar from the Goddess
Makes a luscious peach colored smoothie!

- Homemade almond milk ~ 1 cup (recipe is on page 312)
- Orange, peeled ~ 1
- Fresh squeezed lemon juice ~ a dash
- Dried apricots & pitted dates, washed & chopped ~ totaling 1/2 cup
- Mangos, fresh or frozen ~ 1 - 1/12 cup
- Frozen bananas ~ 2
- Macadamia nuts ~ 1/4 cup
- Vanilla bean, chopped ~ 2 inches
- Cardamon seeds, cinnamon & nutmeg, freshly ground ~ to taste (see page 224)
- Pink Himalayan salt or any salt of your choice ~ to taste
- Ice cubes ~ 1 cup
- Purified water ~ as needed for desired consistency

1) Blend the above ingredients.

2) Top this gorgeous peach colored smoothie with sliced almonds, chopped pistachio nuts & fresh mint leaves, if you like.

Variations ~
- Peaches can be used if you don't have access to mangos.
- Add 1 teaspoon of these 4 super foods; flax, chia, hemp & raw cacao nibs for an extra blast of energy!

Tips~

1) Even though it is preferable to soak the almonds for 8 hours, I just soaked them while I was getting all the other ingredients together & it still came out great. So don't let lack of soaking time be a deterrent from making this blissful smoothie. *"Let's not let perfection be the enemy of the good."*

2) I find it easier to blend in stages. So, try blending all the ingredients with the exception of the mangos & ice. Then, add the mangos & ice to the mixture. This makes the process smoother for smoothies! :)

Superfood Oatmeal

- Whole grain steel cut oats or any oatmeal of your choice ~ 1 cup
- Water or plant milk ~ totaling 2 cups
- Flax seeds, chia seeds & hemp seeds ~ 1 teaspoon each
- Chopped pitted dates & raisins ~ to taste
- Almond pecan milk & fresh fruit, if desired

   (Recipe for nut milks is on page 312.)

1) Combine the ingredients in a sauce pan with purified water.

2) Bring to boil, then lower the heat & simmer until the liquid is absorbed to desired consistency.

3) Top with almond pecan milk & fresh fruit such as berries, if you like.

Vanilla Chia Pudding ~ Four simple ingredients

Makes a delicious healthy breakfast or dessert!
It pairs well with homemade granola & fresh fruit.

- Homemade almond milk ~ 2 cups (recipe is on page 312)
- Pitted dates ~ 4 - 5
- Vanilla bean, chopped ~ 2 - 3 inches
- Chia Seeds ~ 1/2 cup

1) Blend the almond milk, dates & vanilla bean in Vitamix or high-powered blender.

2) Pour into a container & stir in chia seeds.

3) Cover & chill in fridge ideally overnight however even a couple hours is still good.

Variations ~

★ Add in a variety of fruits such as oranges, strawberries, blueberries, mangos, star fruits, apricots, peaches, etc.

★ Sprinkle with nuts, shredded coconut or trail mix, if desired.

Recipes for Lunch Options

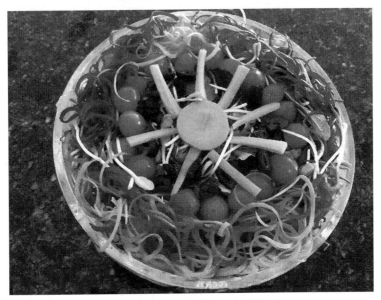

Photo by Meenakshi Angel Honig

Vibrant Rainbow Salad ~ A whole meal & fiesta of vibrant colors in one bowl

Pairs well with chapati flat bread & vegan ricotta 'cheeze'.

A flavorful bed of any vibrant greens such as ~

- ★ Baby lettuce
- ★ Romaine lettuce
- ★ Red leaf lettuce
- ★ Butterhead lettuce
- ★ Green leaf lettuce
- ★ Spinach
- ★ Kale
- ★ Arugula
- ★ Microgreens
- ★ Escarole
- ★ Endive
- ★ Water cress
- ★ Dandelion greens
- ★ Mustard greens
- ★ Collard greens
- ★ Green & purple cabbage

A variety of colorful veggies such as ~

- ★ Carrots
- ★ Beets
- ★ Celery
- ★ Cucumbers
- ★ Tomatoes
- ★ Bell peppers ~ red, green, yellow, orange & purple
- ★ Purple & red onions
- ★ Green onions

A variety of sea vegetables such as ~

- ★ Nori
- ★ Laver
- ★ Kelp
- ★ Wakame
- ★ Hijiki
- ★ Arame

A variety of cooked mushrooms such as ~

- ★ White Button
- ★ Reishi
- ★ Shiitake
- ★ Oyster
- ★ Chanterelle
- ★ Porcini

A variety of fresh sprouts such as ~

- ★ Alfalfa
- ★ Sunflower
- ★ Broccoli
- ★ Daikon radish
- ★ Mung bean
- ★ Lentil sprouts

A variety of olives ~

Olives, ahhhhh! I was so surprised to learn that olives are actually a high-fat fruit!

I never thought of them that way, did you? (If you did, would you please send me an email at angel@angelyoga.com? I would be interested to hear from you!)

Olives are loaded with beneficial compounds. According to a deep mythological history, olives were a gift to humankind from the Greek goddess Athena. There are hundreds of varieties grown throughout the world & they all have a unique appearance & flavor. My 3 favorites are ~

★ Organic Sunfood pitted Peruvian black botija olives

★ Organic Divina pitted green olives

★ Organic Divina kalamata olives

A variety of nuts & seeds such as ~

★ Pine nuts

★ Hazel nuts ~ finely chopped

★ Pecan nuts ~ finely chopped

★ Walnuts ~ finely chopped

★ Sprouted pumpkin seeds

★ Sprouted sunflower seeds

★ Hemp seeds

A variety of fresh herbs such as ~

- ★ Parsley ~ Italian & curly
- ★ Cilantro
- ★ Dill
- ★ Basil
- ★ Oregano
- ★ Fresh garlic
- ★ Tarragon
- ★ Chives
- ★ Mint
- ★ Rosemary

1) Wash greens & herbs & spin dry in a salad spinner.

2) Wash all the other veggies & chop into bitesize 'peaces'.

3) Place your bed of fresh greens in a large bowl.

4) Add the colorful veggies ~ Spiralize carrots, beets & cucumbers for a fun festive touch.

5) Add sprouts, sea vegetables, mushrooms & olives.

6) Add chopped fresh herbs.

7) Add purple onions, green onions & a clove of pressed garlic, if you like.

8) Drizzle with homemade creamy dressing.

9) Top with sauerkraut & sprinkle with nuts & seeds. (Recipes for dressings start on page 270 & the recipe for Sauerkraut is on page 287.)

Fulfilling Buddha Bowls ~ A complete meal & edible rainbow in one bowl

- ★ Any whole grain
- ★ Any bean or legume
- ★ Any assortment of colorful veggies such as ~
- ★ Bell peppers ~ red, yellow, orange, green & purple
- ★ Tomatoes ~ red, yellow & purple
- ★ Beets ~ burgundy, yellow, red & candy striped
- ★ Carrots ~ orange & purple
- ★ Cabbage ~ green, red & purple
- ★ Onions ~ green, yellow, white, red & purple
- ★ Sea veggies such as nori, arame, hijiki, laver or wakame
- ★ Flavor bursting green & black olives
- ★ Cooked mushrooms
- ★ Sprouts & microgreens in rainbow colors
- ★ Fresh chopped herbs
- ★ Crunchy seeds & nuts
- ★ Sauerkraut (recipe is on page 287)
- ★ Homemade creamy dressing, guacamole, pesto or peanut sauce (These recipes start on page 270.)

1) Layer a delicious, artistic & colorful array of the above ingredients in one bowl.

2) Play with a variety of textures such as crisp, creamy, soft, firm & crunchy.

3) Incorporate different shapes such as spirals, cubes, rounds, sticks, grated & julienned.

4) Experiment with different temperatures & food preparation methods such as raw, dehydrated, steamed, grilled, roasted, sautéed, toasted & air fried.

5) Balance the flavors of the 7 tastes ~ bitter, sweet, salty, sour, astringent, pungent & umami.

6) Top with sauerkraut, sprouts, crunchy nuts & seeds.

7) Drizzle with homemade creamy dressing such as, cashew macadamia nut, guacamole, pesto or peanut sauce.

My go-to combo is Texmati rice, which is similar to Basmati rice but grown in Texas, pinto beans & rainbow salad topped with guacamole. (Guacamole recipe is on page 279.)

Experiment & create your favorite go-to Buddha bowl!

Tips ~
1) When I cook grains, I add coriander seeds, fenugreek seeds, cumin seeds & one sheet of washed Kombu sea vegetable. This gives it a savory flavor, adds nutritional value & can also help to promote weight loss.

Coriander Seeds ~ are rich with anti-inflammatory & antibacterial properties. They help to stimulate digestive enzymes & juices, which helps to enhance the digestive system.

Fenugreek Seeds ~ can do wonders for weight loss, diabetes management & liver health. They also help to cut down water-retention & bloating.

Cumin Seeds ~ This earthy spice is very effective in boosting digestion. Cumin helps to fortify the digestive tract & relieves nausea, bloating & constipation. Thymol, an active compound present in cumin, helps to stimulate enzymes that facilitate better secretion of digestive juices. Good digestion promotes better metabolism that leads to healthy weight loss.

2) When preparing grains for your Buddha bowls, remember to avoid using the same old, same old grains, such as rice. Instead, experiment with new options such as buckwheat, spelt, farro & kamut. Different grains have different nutrients & it is beneficial to rotate them.

Variation ~ Try this blend ~

★ Spelt ~ 1/2 cup

★ Farro ~ 1/2 cup

★ Kamut ~ 1/2 cup

★ Coriander seeds, Fenugreek seeds, Cumin seeds ~ a generous pinch of each

★ Kombu sea vegetable ~ 1 sheet washed

★ Pink Himalayan sea salt ~ 3 generous pinches

1) Wash & rinse grains & place them in rice cooker

2) Add 6 cups of water (these grains are very firm & chewy)

3) Add the coriander, fenugreek, cumin, kombu & salt

4) Set the rice cooker for brown rice & press 'play'

Tip ~

When the rice cooker turns off, if the grain is still too firm, add more water & reset on the brown rice setting until desired texture.

Ziggy's Zalad

Pairs well with flatbread & potato pancakes

What I love about Ziggy's Zalad is that it has no dressing, per se, & yet it tastes so flavorful when the veggies marinate in their own natural juices, along with the salt & pepper. It is truly amazing how the absence of a salad dressing is not at all missed in this zestful zalad! It is highly requested for potlucks & is the first to disappear!

- ★ Carrots ~ 2 - 3
- ★ Beets, lightly steamed ~ 2
- ★ Parsnips ~ 3
- ★ Bell Peppers ~ red, yellow, orange & green ~ 1 each
- ★ Radishes ~ red, purple & black ~ to taste
- ★ Turnip ~ 1
- ★ Cucumbers ~ 2
- ★ Tomatoes ~ 3 - 4
- ★ Hazel Nuts ~ a handful
- ★ Pine Nuts ~ a handful
- ★ Sunflower Seeds ~ a handful
- ★ Peanuts ~ a handful
- ★ Cashews ~ a handful
- ★ Walnuts ~ a handful
- ★ Raisins ~ a handful
- ★ Dill ~ 1 bunch
- ★ Parsley (Italian &/or curly) ~ 1 - 2 bunches
- ★ Cilantro ~ 1 bunch
- ★ Green Onion ~1 bunch
- ★ Garlic cloves ~ 3
- ★ Pink Himalayan salt & pepper, freshly ground ~ to taste

1) Cut up all veggies in your own unique style.

2) Add nuts, salt & pepper.

3) Mix & enjoy.

Zoodles with Avocado Pesto Dressing
- ★ Zucchinis ~ 6 medium
- ★ Arugula 1~ cup
- ★ Holy basil ~ 2 cups
- ★ Pine Nuts & Macadamia nuts ~ 1/4 cup each
- ★ Avocado ~ 1 large
- ★ Lemon ~ 1/2 juiced
- ★ Garlic cloves ~ 1 - 2
- ★ Pink Himalayan salt ~ to taste
- ★ Hemp Seeds & basil leaves for garnishing

1) Spriralize 5 zucchinis to make raw zoodles & place in a bowl.

2) Blend the remaining zucchini & other ingredients (except hemp seeds) into a pesto consistency.

3) Stir this mixture evenly into the zoodles.

4) Sprinkle with hemp seeds & garnish with fresh basil leaves.

Romaine Rolls & Love Boats

★ Romaine lettuce or any lettuce that you have on hand
★ Tomatoes
★ Carrots
★ Cucumbers
★ Chopped bell peppers ~ red, green, yellow, orange, purple
★ Olives
★ Sprouts
★ Hummus ~ (recipe is on page 277)
★ Homemade sauerkraut ~ (recipe is on page 287)

1) Detach the romaine leaves carefully, wash & spin dry in a salad spinner.

2) Wash all the other veggies & sprouts.

3) Chop all the veggies into bitesize 'peaces'.

4) Lay down one romaine leaf, like a tortilla or rice paper & spread hummus on it.

5) Layer all the other veggies & sprouts.

6) Top with homemade sauerkraut. (Recipe is on page 287.)

7) Roll up like a spring roll & enjoy being on a roll with your creativity!

8) If the leaf is not big enough to roll you can make it into a love boat.

Variations ~

★ Use collard greens instead of lettuce.

★ Add other veggies that you have on hand.

★ Replace the hummus with ~

   Guacamole (recipe is on page 279)

   Presto Pesto (recipe is on page 278)

   Ricotta Macadamia Nut 'Cheeze' (recipe is on page 272)

Super Yum, Versatile Sandwich, Taco, Tostada, Wrap, Burrito or 'Mini Pizza'

This is my current favorite lunch, dinner or snack!

1) Make a chapati flatbread. (Recipe is on page 290.)

2) Spread with ricotta macadamia nut cheeze. (Recipe is on page 272.)

3) Spread cilantro coconut chutney on top of the ricotta. (Recipe is on page 282.)

4) Cover with rainbow salad. (Recipe is on page 246.)

5) Top with sauerkraut. (Recipe is on page 287.)

6) Cut chapati in half for a sandwich or fold in half like a taco, wrap like a burrito or enjoy open face like a tostada or 'mini pizza'.

Variations ~

- ★ Add cooked beans such as pinto, red chili beans, kidney beans, adzuki beans, etc.
- ★ Add salsa.
- ★ Replace ricotta macadamia nut cheeze with other non-dairy cheezes.
- ★ Add guacamole. (Recipe is on page 279.)
- ★ Add presto pesto. (Recipe is on page 278.)
- ★ Add hummus. (Recipe is on page 277.)
- ★ Add falafel. (Recipe is on page 262.)

Recipes for Dinner Options

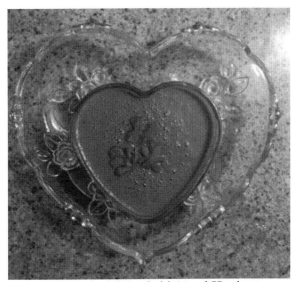

Photo by Meenakshi Angel Honig

Creamy Vibrant Green Comfort Soup

Even though I lean toward raw food, there are those times on a chilly or rainy evening, that I just really feel like having something hot, like soup. Here is a quick & easy recipe that I came up with, which is one of my favorite blended soups. In just a few minutes you have this hot, creamy, gorgeous green, yummy blended soup that is so nourishing & comforting!

- ★ Potatoes ~ 2 medium
- ★ Kale &/or spinach ~ large handful
- ★ Cashews, pine nuts, macadamia nuts, or any combination thereof ~ totaling 3/4 cup
- ★ Hemp seeds ~ a few tablespoons
- ★ Red chili pepper or jalapeño ~ 1 (deseeded, unless you like it hot!)

- ★ Garlic cloves ~ 2 - 3
- ★ Chopped green onion ~ 1 stalk
- ★ Fresh herbs such as basil, thyme, cilantro, parsley, dill & oregano ~ to taste
- ★ Pink Himalayan sea salt or salt of your choice ~ to taste
- ★ Lime ~ a squeeze
- ★ Sprouted sunflower seeds to garnish

1) Wash, chop & steam potatoes until tender.

2) Add potatoes to the Vitamix with the water that you steamed them in.

3) Add the other ingredients, except the sprouted sunflower seeds & lime, & blend.

4) Add more water, if needed, to get smooth, creamy consistency.

5) Place in bowl, add a squeeze of lime & top with sprouted sunflower seeds.

Variation ~
- ★ The potato & nuts are what make it creamy. For variety, replace the kale & spinach with broccoli, green beans, swiss chard, dandelion greens, corn, or whatever vegetables you are drawn to.

Fabulous Falafel

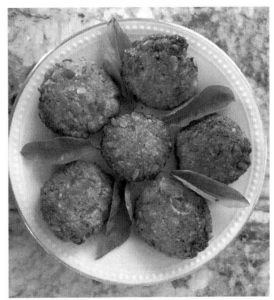

Photo by Meenakshi Angel Honig

I will be the first to admit that my *unprocessed* version of falafel in no way compares to the "real deal". However, if we step out of the realm of comparisons for a moment & evaluate it on its own merit, it's super yum!

I fell in love with falafel at a young age & it became one of my favorite foods when I was visiting Israel. When I shifted to an unprocessed diet, the thought of never having falafel again was a daunting idea. So, I created my own unprocessed version & here it is!

Please keep in mind that every batch is unique depending on what ingredients I have on hand. You can play with it, adding & deleting as you like. Stay creative! As long as you use good ingredients, keep it to a consistency that sticks together & infuse it with love, it's going to be great!

I personally do not use anything from a can but you 'can' if you like. Or you can 'can' that idea & use the dry garbanzo beans, as I do.

Garbanzo beans, also known as chickpeas, are a rich source of vitamins, minerals & fiber. Chickpeas offer a variety of health benefits, such as improving digestion, aiding weight management & reducing the risk of several diseases.

I love to make falafel for special occasions. It also makes a great protein-packed snack to have on hand. It is super easy to pack for a snack on the go & perfect for picnics. It is also fabulous for a gourmet dinner when served on flatbread with rainbow salad, sauerkraut & drizzled with lemon tahini dressing!

Recipes for the whole ensemble are all included in this book!

- ★ Flatbread recipe is on page 289.
- ★ Rainbow Salad recipe is on page 246.
- ★ Sauerkraut recipe is on page 287.
- ★ Lemon Tahini Dressing recipe is on page 273.

- ★ Dry Garbanzo beans, soaked ~ 1 1/2 cups (after soaking)
- ★ Hemp seeds ~ 1/4 cup
- ★ Macadamia nuts ~ 1/2 cup
- ★ Sprouted sunflower seeds ~ 1/4 cup
- ★ Spelt & or garbanzo flour, freshly ground in Vitamix or coffee/seed grinder ~ 1/4 cup
- ★ Lemon juice, freshly squeezed ~ 1 1/2
- ★ Parsley, Italian &/or curly, fresh ~ 1/4 cup

- ★ Cilantro, fresh, destemmed ~ 1/4 cup
- ★ Dill, fresh ~ 1/4 cup
- ★ Garlic cloves ~ 3 - 4
- ★ Red chili pepper ~ 1 (deseeded unless you like it hot!)
- ★ Coriander seeds, fenugreek seeds, cumin seeds ~ a pinch of each
- ★ Pink Himalayan sea salt or any salt of your choice ~ to taste
- ★ Purified water ~ as needed to process in food processor

1) Wash & soak dry garbanzo beans in purified water. (Although it is ideal to soak beans overnight or for 8 hours, a shorter time is still beneficial, so let's not let perfection be the enemy of the good.)

2) Drain & rinse garbanzo beans & place all the ingredients in a food processor.

3) Process until it is a cohesive mixture. (Do not over process or it will become like hummus.)

4) Refrigerate mixture to make it firmer. (optional)

5) Roll into balls, flatten like a disc & place on parchment paper. (If the mixture is too loose to roll into balls, stir in more flour, sunflower seeds & hemp seeds to thicken it up.)

6) Bake in air fryer at 370° for approximately 8 minutes on each side or until desired crispiness. If you do not have an air fryer, line a pan with parchment paper & bake in pre-heated oven at 350° for approximately 8 minutes on each side or until evenly baked & crisp.

7) Serve with a lemon tahini dipping sauce garnished with chopped fresh parsley, cilantro & mint.

Air French Fries

★ Potatoes ~ 2

★ Homemade creamy dressing (recipes start on page 270)

★ Pink Himalayan salt & black pepper, freshly ground ~ to taste

1) Wash & slice potatoes in strips like French fries & place in mixing bowl.

2) Coat with homemade creamy dressing.

3) Season with salt & pepper.

4) Place on parchment paper in air fryer or in toaster oven for about 9 minutes on each side or until crispy brown.

5) Enjoy with the dipping sauce of your choice. (Recipes start on page 270.)

Variations ~

- ★ Coat with other dressings such as cashew blended with sun-dried tomato or pesto sauce.
- ★ Add sliced red onions, chopped fresh garlic & hemps seeds in with the potato mixture.
- ★ Replace potatoes with cauliflower or breadfruit.

Vegetable Dhal with Basmati Rice

- ★ Red lentils ~ 3/4 cup
- ★ Split yellow peas ~ 1/4 cup
- ★ Split green peas ~ 1/4 cup
- ★ Onion ~ 1
- ★ Garlic cloves ~ 4 - 6
- ★ Carrots ~ 2
- ★ Celery ~ 2 stalks
- ★ Green beans, chopped ~ 1 cup
- ★ Potatoes, chopped ~ 1
- ★ Kale &/or spinach, chopped ~ large handful
- ★ Coriander seeds, fenugreek seeds & cumin seeds ~ a generous pinch of each
- ★ Chili pepper or jalapeño pepper ~ 1 (deseeded unless you like it hot!)
- ★ Fresh turmeric ~ 3/4 teaspoon minced
- ★ Fresh ginger ~ 3/4 teaspoon minced
- ★ Purified water ~ about 6 cups or more

1) Soak the red lentils, split yellow peas & split green peas in a large pot. (It is preferable to soak for a few hours but less time also works well, so let's not let perfection be the enemy of good.)

2) Drain & rinse several times.

3) Add about 3 times as much purified water as the legumes. (Use more water if you want it like a soup & less water if you want it like a veggie stew.)

4) Add coriander, fenugreek, cumin, Himalayan sea salt & deseeded chili pepper or deseeded jalapeño pepper.

5) Bring to a boil & then lower the heat to simmer.

6) Wash & chop all of the veggies & add to the pot.

7) Add the minced ginger & turmeric to the pot.

8) Simmer all of the ingredients until tender.

9) Serve with Basmati rice or quinoa.

10) Garnish with freshly chopped parsley & cilantro.

Variations ~
* Add any other veggies that you have on hand such as broccoli, zucchini, turnips, etc.
* Adding chopped beets or tomatoes gives it a rich golden red color.
* Adding tamarind paste from the pod, gives it a rich sweet & sour flavor.

A Medley of Steamed Veggies drizzled with Peanut Macadamia Nut Sauce

Pairs well with rice, millet & quinoa

Any veggies that you like such as ~

★ Broccoli

★ Cauliflower

★ Green beans

★ Beets

★ Carrots

★ Cabbage

★ Potatoes

★ Red Onions

★ Garlic

★ Nuts, finely chopped ~ to garnish.

★ Parsley, sage, rosemary & thyme ~ to garnish.

1) Wash & chop veggies.

2) Steam until tender.

3) Place in bowl & drizzle with peanut macadamia nut sauce. (Recipe is on page 285.)

4) Garnish with finely chopped nuts & freshly chopped parsley, sage, rosemary & thyme.

Angel Hair 'Pasta' with Pesto Sauce

★ Spaghetti Squash ~ 1

★ Presto Pesto Sauce (recipe is on page 278)

★ Raw sprouted pumpkin seeds ~ to garnish

1) Cut a spaghetti squash in half, remove seeds & steam until tender.

2) Scrape out the spaghetti squash with a fork so that it looks like angel hair pasta & place on a plate.

3) Cover with pesto sauce & garnish with sprouted pumpkin seeds.

Tip ~

1) Cut the spaghetti squash in half & salt it. Let it sit for 15 - 20 minutes to draw out the moisture before steaming it. Less moisture makes for less mushy noodles.

Variation ~

★ Replace the pesto sauce with marinara sauce or peanut sauce.
(Recipe for peanut macadamia nut sauce is on page 285.)

Recipes for Dressings, Dips, 'Cheeze', Sauces, Gravy, Nut butters, Chutney & Sauerkraut

Creamy Cashew/Macadamia Nut Dressing & Dip

Many people have commented that if they had this dressing, it would make it easy for them to go vegan & oil free. The only oil in it is what occurs naturally in the nuts.

* Cashews ~ 1 cup
* Macadamia nuts ~ 1/2 cup
* Pine nuts ~ 1/2 cup
* Lime or lemon juice, freshly squeezed ~ 1 medium (or you can use the whole lime or lemon, peeled & deseeded, if you prefer)
* Chili pepper ~ 1 - 2 (deseeded unless you like it hot, or omit if you prefer no heat)
* Garlic cloves, chopped ~ 2
* Pink Himalayan sea salt, freshly ground or any salt of your choice ~ to taste
* Purified water ~ as needed for desired consistency

1) Soak the nuts in a bowl while you are getting the other ingredients in the Vitamix, high-powered blender or food processor.

2) Rinse & drain the nuts & add them to the blender.

3) Blend to desired consistency.

Tips ~

1) Add more water for salad dressing & less water for dip or 'cheeze'.

2) Blend more for a creamy consistency & blend less for a chunky texture.

3) If you are not going to use all the dressing right away, place half of it in a freezer-safe container & freeze. Then pull it out & defrost, when desired. This helps the dressing to stay fresh longer.

Variations ~

Add any of the following ingredients to the basic recipe ~

★ Replace the macadamia & pine nuts with cashews, making all the nuts cashew.

★ Additional pine nuts & fresh basil for a pesto flavor

★ Soaked & rinsed sun-dried tomatoes & fresh tomatoes for a "Thousand Island" flavor

★ Fresh herbs such as basil, dill, oregano, chives, thyme, tarragon, cilantro & parsley

★ Fresh green onions

★ Tamarind ~ Remove the reddish-brown colored paste from the seeds in the pod & add the paste to the blender for a sweet/sour, rich base note flavor.

★ Green pitted olives, etc…. Just let your imagination take you for a joy ride!

Ricotta Macadamia Nut 'Cheeze'

Pairs well with chapati, lentil flatbread & cilantro chutney

This is my new favorite 'cheeze.' I learned how to make this simple & delicious macadamia nut 'cheeze' from my friend Ricardo, so I call it *Ricardo Ricotta*." It can be used like ricotta or spread like cream cheese. It is very versatile & super yum!

- ★ Macadamia nuts, dry roasted & salted ~ 1 1/2 cups
- ★ Lemon juice, freshly squeezed ~ approximately 5 tablespoons
- ★ Garlic cloves ~ 2 - 3
- ★ Red chili peppers ~ 1 - 2 (deseeded, unless you like it hot!)
- ★ Pink Himalayan salt or salt of your choice, freshly ground ~ to taste
- ★ Purified water ~ as needed to for desired consistency

1) Add the ingredients to a food processor & press play. Pause the processor & scrape down the sides, as needed. Process until it is a white, fluffy, creamy consistency.

2) Add more lemon juice or water, as needed, for flavor & consistency.

Variation ~

- ★ Add fresh herbs such as chives, cilantro, basil, rosemary & oregano.

Lemon Tahini Dressing & Dip

This is great as a salad dressing or use it to make sesame gravy.

When paired with falafel, it is a marriage made in heaven! Open sesame!

Sesame seeds are power packed with health benefits! They are rich in copper, manganese, magnesium & calcium, all of which contribute to good bone health.

Just 2 tablespoons of sesame seeds provide about 4 grams of fiber. Research shows that adding more fiber to your diet may lower blood pressure, improve blood cholesterol levels, reduce inflammation & help to control diabetes.

Sesame seeds are loaded with antioxidant-rich phytosterols, which are beneficial plant compounds, that have been scientifically shown to lower cholesterol. Having lower cholesterol levels leads to other benefits, such as a reduced risk of heart attacks & strokes & helps to protect against the development of certain cancers.

Sesame seeds also provide healthy fats, such as mono & polyunsaturated fats. These healthy fats help the body absorb nutrients & vitamins, such as A, D, E & K, that are vital for good vision, strong bones & nerve development. They also help regulate hormones, body temperature & contribute to radiant skin, strong nails & healthy hair!

- ★ Sesame seeds ~ 1/2 cup
- ★ Pine nuts ~ 1/4 cup
- ★ Macadamia nuts ~ 1/4 cup
- ★ Lemon juice, freshly squeezed ~ 1 medium
- ★ Garlic ~ 3 cloves
- ★ Red chili pepper ~ 1 (deseeded unless you like it hot!)
- ★ Pink Himalayan sea salt & pepper, freshly ground ~ to taste
- ★ Purified water ~ about 1 1/2 cups or to desired consistency

1) Place the above ingredients in a Vitamix or high-powered blender & blend until creamy.

Tips ~

1) Blends best if you place the lemon juice on the bottom closest to the blades.

2) Use more water for dressing & less water for a thicker dip.

Variations ~

- ★ Add fresh basil, dill or other fresh herbs.
- ★ Add 1/2 red bell pepper for a golden red color.

Green Goddess Avocado Dressing

Makes a vibrant lime green color dressing!

★ Avocado ~ 1

★ Macadamia &/or pine nuts ~ totaling 1/2 cup

★ Lemon or lime juice, freshly squeezed ~ 1

★ Garlic cloves ~ 2

★ Green onions ~ 1 stalk

★ Fresh herbs such as basil, thyme, parsley, cilantro & oregano ~ to taste

★ Red chili pepper or jalapeño ~ 1 (deseeded unless you like it hot!)

★ Pink Himalayan sea salt & pepper, freshly ground ~ to taste

★ Purified water, if needed ~ to desired consistency

1) Scoop out the avocado & place in Vitamix, high powered blender or food processor.

2) Add the other ingredients, blend & enjoy!

Almond Lime Dressing

★ Almonds, soaked ~ 1 cup

★ Hemp seeds ~ 1/4 cup

★ Lime, peeled & deseeded ~ 1/2 - 3/4

★ Garlic cloves ~ 2

★ Red chili pepper ~ 1 (deseeded unless you like it hot!)

★ Pink Himalayan sea salt, freshly ground ~ to taste

★ Purified water ~ as needed for desired consistency

1) Place the above ingredients in a Vitamix or high-powered blender & blend until creamy.

Tips ~

1) Blends best if you place the lime on the bottom closest to the blades.

2) Use more water for dressing & less water for a thicker dip.

Variation ~

★ Add fresh basil &/or other fresh herbs.

Hummus

★ Garbanzo beans, cooked ~ 1 1/2 cup

★ Cumin seeds, whole ~ a generous pinch

★ Pine nuts, cashews, macadamia nuts, sesame seeds, hemp seeds, sprouted sunflower seeds, any or all ~ totaling 3/4 cup

★ Freshly squeezed lemon or lime juice ~ 1

★ Red chili pepper or jalapeño (deseeded unless you like it hot!) ~ to taste

★ Garlic cloves ~ 2 - 3

★ Red bell pepper ~ 1/2 (red pepper makes it a beautiful golden-red color)

★ Pink Himalayan sea salt or any salt of your choice ~ to taste

★ Mint leaves & parsley ~ to garnish

1) Wash dry garbanzo beans (soaking is preferable but not essential).

2) Place in a saucepan & add purified water until twice the volume of the garbanzo beans.

3) Add cumin seeds & pink Himalayan salt.

4) Bring to a boil & then simmer until tender but still firm.

5) Blend the lemon or lime juice, red pepper, garlic, deseeded hot pepper, nuts, seeds & salt.

6) Add the cooked garbanzo beans to the blender with just enough of the liquid that you boiled them in, to blend smoothly. Add additional water, if needed.

7) Garnish with chopped red pepper, mint leaves & parsley.

Tip ~

1) Can also be made in a food processor.

Variations ~

★ Blend fresh herbs such as parsley, basil & cilantro into the hummus.

★ Add green onions.

★ Add olives.

Presto Pesto

★ Pine nuts &/or sprouted sunflower seeds ~ totaling 2 cups
★ Hemp Seeds ~ 1/2 cup
★ Baby spinach ~ 1 cup
★ Fresh basil ~ 2 cups
★ Lemon or lime, freshly squeezed ~ 1 large
★ Garlic cloves ~ 2 - 3
★ Red chili or jalapeño pepper ~ 1 (deseeded unless you like it hot!)
★ Chives, chopped ~ to taste
★ Pink Himalayan salt & pepper, freshly ground ~ to taste
★ Purified water ~ as needed to blend

1) Blend & garnish with fresh basil leaves.

Guacamole

- Ripe avocados ~ 2
- Lime juice, freshly squeezed ~ 1
- Tomatoes, chopped ~ 1/2 cup
- Cilantro, chopped ~ 1/2 cup
- Red onions, finely chopped ~ 1 slice
- Garlic ~ 2 cloves
- Jalapeño pepper (deseeded unless you like it hot!) ~ to taste
- Pink Himalayan salt & pepper, freshly ground ~ to taste

1) Mash ripe avocados in a bowl.

2) Add fresh lime juice, chopped tomatoes, cilantro, red onions, jalapeño, garlic, salt & pepper.

3) Mix thoroughly with Love & garnish with fresh cilantro leaves.

Savory Vegan Gravy

- ★ Red onion sliced thinly ~ 3/4
- ★ Garlic sliced thinly ~ 8 cloves
- ★ Oyster mushrooms chopped, or mushrooms of your choice ~ 1/2 pound
- ★ Fresh ginger, minced ~ 3/4 teaspoon
- ★ Fresh turmeric, minced ~ 3/4 teaspoon
- ★ Fresh rosemary, chopped ~ to taste
- ★ Fresh oregano, chopped ~ to taste
- ★ Red chili pepper ~ 1 (deseeded unless you like it hot!)
- ★ Homemade cashew dressing ~ 1 cup (Recipe is on page 270.)
- ★ Pink Himalayan salt & pepper, freshly ground ~ to taste
- ★ Purified water ~ as needed for desired consistency
- ★ Lemon or lime ~ a squeeze right before serving

1) Sauté the onion, garlic, mushrooms, ginger, turmeric, red chili pepper & chopped fresh rosemary in water, in a large skillet, until soft.

2) Stir in homemade cashew dressing.

3) Add purified water to make it the consistency of gravy.

4) Add a squeeze of lemon or lime right before serving for an extra burst of zestful flavor.

Tip ~

1) Rosemary & oregano are beautiful, medicinal, culinary herbs that are so easy to grow on your deck as potted plants! Then, you can just go out & pick a few sprigs & a few leaves when preparing food.

Rosemary is an aromatic shrub that has a slightly minty, sage-like, peppery, balsamic taste with a woody aftertaste. It is a rich source of antioxidants & anti-inflammatory compounds which help to boost the immune system & improve blood circulation. Rosemary is considered a cognitive stimulant & can help to improve memory. It is also known to boost alertness & focus.

Just wash, de-stem & chop it finely.

Oregano is high in antioxidants & may help fight off bacteria & viruses, potentially reduce the growth of cancer cells & help alleviate inflammation.

Both of these fresh herbs bring a special alive flavor to your cooked dishes & salads!

Variations ~

★ Grind spelt berries or dry garbanzo beans in a seed grinder to make a fresh flour & add to the gravy to make it thicker.

★ Add cooked grain, cooked beans & fresh spinach to the hot gravy & stir. This makes a creamy one-skillet dinner.

★ This gravy can also be used as the base for creamed soups such as cream of broccoli & vegan corn chowder. Super Yum!

- Replace cashew dressing with homemade lemon tahini dressing for a Middle Eastern flavor or peanut macadamia nut sauce for a savory Southeast Asian flair!
  (Recipe for lemon tahini dressing is on page 273 & recipe for peanut macadamia nut sauce is on page 285.)

Cilantro Coconut Chutney

Chutney is a spicy or savory condiment originating in India. Chutney is made from fruits, vegetables, herbs & spices. It's used to provide balance to an array of dishes or highlight a specific flavor profile.

This chutney pops with flavor & is outrageously tasty! It pairs well with chapatis, lentil flatbread, macadamia nut 'cheeze' & stirred into cooked grains.

- Cilantro ~ 1 bunch
- Coconut, dried & unsweetened ~ 1 cup
- Lime juice, freshly squeezed ~ 1
- Jalapeno or red chili (deseeded unless you like it hot!) ~ to taste
- Garlic cloves ~ 2 - 3
- Pink Himalayan salt or salt of your choice, freshly ground ~ to taste
- Purified water ~ as needed for desired consistency

1) Wash & chop fresh cilantro & breathe in the sublime aroma!

2) Chop jalapeño & garlic cloves.

3) Squeeze lime to make fresh lime juice.

4) Place the shredded coconut in the food processor first & process until it is a fine texture.

5) Add all the other ingredients, including the salt, & process to a chutney-like consistency.

6) Pause the processor & scrape down the sides, as needed.

7) Add water or additional lime juice, as needed, for consistency & flavor.

Variation ~

★ Dry roast mustard seeds in a cast iron or non-stick frying pan. Stir into chutney after it is processed to add texture & flavor.

Nut Butters

According to the FDA (Food & Drug Administration) *Food Defect Levels Handbook*, commercial peanut butter may contain insect fragments, rodent's hairs, excreta & other filth. Most commercial peanut butter also includes added oil, sugar & preservatives.

This can all be avoided by making your own from whole, clean nuts. I am astounded by how quick & easy it is to make your own fresh, delicious nut butters in about 5 minutes with a food processor! I wish I had known this earlier in my life! Glad we know it now!

Peanut Macadamia Nut Butter

Pairs well with apples, celery & flatbread
(Flatbread recipe is on page 289.)

- ★ Raw unsalted peanuts ~ 2 cups
- ★ Dry roasted, salted macadamia nuts ~ 1 cup
- ★ Medjool Dates ~ 2 - 3 pitted

1) Place the ingredients in a food processor & process until creamy!

Super simple, super fast & super delicious!

Tip ~

1) Process more for creamier nut butter & process less for chunkier nut butter.

Variation ~

- ★ Replace the macadamia nuts with other high oil content nuts such as Brazil nuts, pecans & hazel nuts.

Peanut Macadamia Nut Sauce

This sauce is great drizzled over a medley of steamed veggies. It pairs well with quinoa, rice or millet.

* Nut butter ~ 1 1/2 cups (recipe on page 285)
* Raw unsalted peanuts ~ 1 cup
* Garlic ~ 2 - 3 cloves
* Freshly squeezed lime juice ~ 1
* Red chili pepper ~ 1 (deseeded unless you like it super hot!)
* Pink Himalayan salt ~ to taste
* Water ~ as needed for desired consistency

1) Place the nut butter in a Vitamix or high-powered blender with the lime juice, garlic cloves, chili pepper, salt & water.

2) Blend until creamy.

3) Then add the peanuts & blend on very low speed so they blend in but are still a bit crunchy to provide texture for the peanut sauce.

Variation ~

* Add tamarind paste from the pod for a rich sweet/sour flavor.

Cashew Cream

It is great on top of waffles, fresh fruit pies & parfaits in place of whipped cream.

- ★ Raw cashews ~ 2 cups
- ★ Medjool dates, pitted ~ 3 - 4
- ★ Vanilla bean ~ 2 inches
- ★ Lemon juice ~ a squeeze
- ★ Pink Himalayan salt ~ to taste
- ★ Purified water ~ as needed for desired consistency

1) Soak raw cashews & medjool dates.

2) Make sure to drain the liquid after soaking & discard it.

3) Place in blender & add chopped vanilla bean.

4) Add squeeze of lemon juice & pinch of salt.

5) Add purified water & blend to the consistency similar to non-dairy yogurt.

Tip ~

1) You can soak the cashews & dates for as little as an hour but overnight is best because soaking them pulls out the phytic acid & enzyme inhibitors, making the cream tastier, easier to digest & giving it a more velvety consistency.

Sauerkraut

Beneficial probiotics, or 'live bacteria', are produced in the fermentation process of making sauerkraut. These probiotics are what give sauerkraut most of its health benefits. Sauerkraut is a great source of dietary fiber, vitamins C & K, potassium, calcium & phosphorus.

According to *NurseMary.com* sauerkraut contains far more lactobacillus than yogurt, making it a superior source of this probiotic. Most canned sauerkraut has been pasteurized, which kills off the good bacteria, so it provides more health benefits if you make it yourself. Sauerkraut makes a flavorful condiment for salads, wraps & Buddha bowls.

- ★ Green cabbage ~ 1 small
- ★ Purple cabbage ~ 1 small
- ★ Carrots ~ 3 - 4
- ★ Onion, red or purple ~ 1
- ★ Garlic cloves ~ 8
- ★ Ginger, freshly minced ~ 1 teaspoon
- ★ Turmeric, freshly minced ~ 1 teaspoon
- ★ Cilantro ~1 cup
- ★ Italian parsley ~ 1 cup
- ★ Dill &/or any other fresh herbs such as oregano & rosemary ~ to taste
- ★ Red chili pepper or jalapeño pepper ~ 1 - 2 (deseeded, unless you like it hot!)
- ★ Pink Himalayan salt or salt of your choice ~ 2 tablespoons

(Do not use less than 2 tablespoons of salt because it is vital for the fermentation process.)

1) Wash & chop the ingredients into bite size pieces, or shred in a food processor & place in a large bowl (or 2 bowls, if needed).

2) Stir in 2 tablespoons of pink Himalayan salt.

3) Use tamper from Vitamix to stir & stomp down the veggies so the liquid from the veggies releases, when combined with the salt. This is the brining solution that will cover your veggies when you put them in a clean jar to ferment.

4) Leave the mixture to sit for a while so that the veggies continue to release their liquid. You can expedite the release of the natural liquids by kneading the veggies with clean hands. Remember that your hands are wands of light, so consciously use them to infuse love & mantras into your food.

5) When there is enough liquid to cover the veggies completely, pack them tightly into a clean mason jar with a lid. Make sure that the veggies are ***completely*** submerged in the liquid as it must be anaerobic (without oxygen), or it can become toxic.

6) Place a bowl under the jar to catch any liquid that may emerge from the jar as it is fermenting & place the jar in a cool place such as in kitchen pantry or cabinet.

7) Let it ferment for a few days & then, voila, you have delicious homemade sauerkraut packed with natural probiotics!

Recipes for Flatbreads ~ A Whole New World!

OK friends, it took me 67 years to discover what I am about to offer you & it opened up a whole new culinary world for me! In fact, when I discovered this, I literally went to YouTube & played the theme song from Aladdin entitled, *A Whole New World*, sung by Peabo Bryson & Regina Belle, to dance & celebrate!!

Just to put this discovery in context, as I mentioned before, I became a vegetarian around the age of 11. Then, I became a vegan in 1987 inspired by a handout based on the book, *Diet for a New America*, by John Robbins. When I had a life-changing conversation with Ryan Earhart in 2017 & realized the disgusting debris that goes into processed food, I spiraled up to the next level & chose an ***unprocessed*** vegan diet.

So since 2017, I have eaten only *unprocessed* or *minimally processed* food. This has excluded all products made with commercially ground flour & spices, sugar, oil, etc., in addition, of course, to no meat, eggs, dairy or fish. Just to clarify, this is not a deprivation, it is a choice that leads to a higher level of wellbeing on both physical & spiritual levels.

So given that context, you can imagine how excited I am to have discovered that I can make my own clean, freshly ground flour in a Vitamix or coffee/seed grinder in a minute or so!

Once I discovered that, it opened up a whole new culinary world for me because now I can make my own unprocessed flat breads & other recipes that call for flour with this 'flowering' awareness! I am thoroughly enjoying my first "bread" in over 4 years!

Here are a few of my favorite new recipes with freshly ground flour!

Chapati Flat Bread

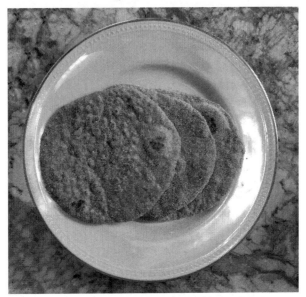

Photo by Meenakshi Angel Honig

This flat bread has just 3 ingredients!
It is so simple, delicious, satisfying & versatile!

It pairs well with ricotta macadamia nut "cheeze,' cilantro coconut chutney, guacamole, hummus, presto pesto, falafel & homemade peanut butter.
(All of these recipes are included in the recipe section of this book!)

★ Spelt berries, freshly ground ~ 1 cup

★ Purified water, warm ~ as needed for dough consistency

★ Pink Himalayan salt, freshly ground or salt of your choice ~ to taste

1) Grind spelt berries in a Vitamix or coffee/seed grinder into a fine flour & place in a mixing bowl. (It just takes a minute or so to make fresh flour!)

2) Warm purified water (not hot, just lukewarm).

3) Little by little, add the water to the flour, kneading it with your clean hands until it becomes a dough-like consistency. (Your hands are wands of light. Remember to consciously infuse mantras & love into the food that you are preparing.)

4) Roll the dough into a ball or log & place in the bowl.

5) Cover with a clean, moist towel & let it rest for about 15 minutes.

6) Pre-heat an eco-friendly, non-stick griddle to 350°.

7) Take a small "peace" of the dough about the size of a lemon, roll into a ball & flatten like a disc.

8) On a lightly floured surface, with a lightly floured rolling pin to avoiding sticking, roll the disc into a tortilla/chapati shape.

9) Using a spatula, place the chapati onto the pre-heated, non-stick griddle.

10) Cook for about a minute on each side or until desired crispiness.

Variations ~

★ Add whole sesame seeds to the dough.

★ Replace the spelt flour with freshly ground raw buckwheat groats, rye berries, wheat berries, brown rice, garbanzo beans, oats, or any combination thereof, to make a variety of different flours. Experiment & find your favorite combos!

★ Add finely chopped fresh herbs such as chives, cilantro, basil, rosemary & oregano.

★ Add finely chopped olives, jalapeño, garlic & onions.

Tip ~

1) I keep a toothbrush designated to be a nail brush in my kitchen. When I am going to be kneading dough with my hands, I wash them thoroughly & use the nail brush to clean underneath my nails before starting.

Lentil Flat Bread

Miraculously simple & yummy!

★ Red lentils ~ 1 cup

★ Purified water ~ 1 cup, or more as needed for desired consistency

★ Fenugreek, cumin & coriander seeds ~ a pinch of each

★ Pink Himalayan salt or salt of your choice ~ to taste

1) Wash red lentils thoroughly & let soak in water for a few hours.

2) Drain the soaking water & rinse.

3) Add the red lentils, purified water, seeds & salt to a Vitamix or blender.

4) Blend until a creamy, batter-like consistency.

5) Pre-heat an eco-friendly, non-stick griddle to 350°.

6) Pour batter, like a pancake, onto the griddle.

7) Cook for about a minute on each side or to desired crispiness.

Variations ~

★ Replace red lentils with brown or green lentils.
★ Add whole sesame seeds to the batter.

Potato Pancakes

Super simple & super delicious!

There are more than 200 varieties of potatoes sold throughout the US. Each of these varieties fit into one of seven potato type categories: russet, red, white, yellow, blue/purple, fingerling & petite. Experiment with different kinds of potatoes & discover your favorites!

- ★ Potatoes ~ 1 cup
- ★ Oat flour, freshly ground ~ 1 cup
- ★ Pink Himalayan salt or salt of your choice, freshly ground ~ to taste

1) Wash, peel if needed, & chop potatoes.

2) Place in steamer & steam until soft.

3) Grind oats into fresh flour in a Vitamix or coffee/seed grinder. (It just takes a minute or so.)

4) Combine flour & warm soft potatoes in a bowl.

5) Knead together with your clean hands into dough & form into a ball or log.

6) Pre-heat eco-friendly, non-stick griddle to 350°.

7) Take a "peace" of the dough, about the size of a lime. Roll it into a ball & flatten like a disk.

8) Lightly coat your surface & rolling pin with a little of the oat flour to prevent sticking & roll into the shape of a pancake.

9) Using a spatula, place pancake on the pre-heated griddle & cook for about a minute on each side or until desired crispness.

Variations ~

★ Experiment with different kinds of potatoes.
★ Add finely chopped olives, garlic, onions, red chili or jalapeño.
★ Add fresh chopped herbs such as rosemary, oregano, chives, thyme, dill & basil.

Recipes for Healthy & Sumptuous Snacks

Crispy Roasted Garbanzo Beans

* Garbanzo beans, dry ~ 1 cup
* Cumin seeds ~ a pinch
* Your choice of homemade salad dressing ~ to coat thoroughly (recipes start on page 270)
* Pink Himalayan salt & pepper, freshly ground ~ to taste

1) Wash dry garbanzo beans ~ soaking is preferable but not essential.

2) Place in a saucepan & add purified water until twice the volume of the garbanzo beans.

3) Add the cumin seeds, pink Himalayan sea salt & cook until tender but still firm.

4) Drain liquid & reserve for other recipes such as vegan gravy.

5) Place the drained garbanzo beans in a bowl & sprinkle with salt & pepper.

6) Coat with homemade dressing.

7) Roast in Air fryer for 8 minutes then stir & roast for about 6 minutes, or longer if you like them more crispy.

8) If you do not have an Air fryer (which I love because you can make food crispy without any added oil) then line a baking sheet with parchment paper, distribute evenly & bake at 400° for about 16 minutes, stirring half way through.

Enjoy this delicious, crispy, high protein snack that is great to have on hand for a quick pick-me-up!

Variation ~
- Stir in chopped garlic & hot peppers when coating the garbanzo beans with dressing.

Presto Pesto Popcorn

Popcorn is high in fiber & is also a good source of polyphenols, which are antioxidants that have been linked to better blood circulation & digestive health, as well as a potentially lower risk of certain cancers. Another health benefit of popcorn is its high satiety.

- Popcorn
- Presto Pesto dressing or cashew dressing (Recipes start on page 270.)
- Pink Himalayan salt & pepper, freshly ground

1) Air pop the popcorn.

2) Coat with pesto or cashew dressing.

3) Sprinkle with salt & pepper to taste.

Delicious, filling & fun!

Avocado "Toast"

This is one of my favorite snacks or it can be a meal in itself!

- Chapati Flatbread ~ 1 (recipe is on page 290)
- Avocado, ripe ~ 1
- Black Himalayan sea salt, freshly ground or salt of your choice ~ to taste

1) Make a chapati flatbread. (Recipe is on page 290.)

2) Mash a ripe avocado with a fork.

3) Spread the avocado on the chapati & sprinkle with black Himalayan salt.

Variations ~

- Add some lemon juice, minced garlic & finely chopped red chili to the mashed avocado.
- Top avocado with sliced tomatoes, arugula, chopped basil leaves & chopped olives.
- Top avocado with rainbow salad & homemade sauerkraut. (Recipes are on pages 246 & 287.)
- Be creative & find your own favorite combos!

Recipes for Desserts

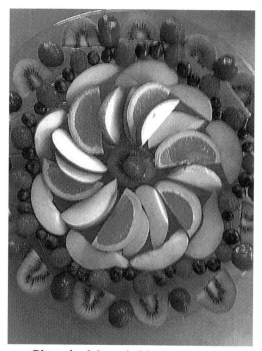

Photo by Meenakshi Angel Honig

Frozen cherries, strawberries, blueberries

Pure & simple! ~ A delicious, healthy replacement for ice cream & free of all the added sugar & other junk!

1) Wash frozen fruit & place in a bowl.

2) Allow to defrost for a few minutes until semi-frozen & enjoy!

As Leonardo da Vinci said, *"Simplicity is the ultimate sophistication."*

And as Meenakshi Angel Honig said, *"Simplicity is felicity!"*

Variations ~

★ Frozen mango, pineapple & other fruits are also great healthy, delicious substitutes for ice cream.

★ Top with chopped nuts & shredded coconut.

★ For a special fun treat, freeze grapes & float them in a plastic bowl in a hot tub or in your bathtub for a cool, refreshing & delicious dessert!

Fruit Salad

Makes a great breakfast or dessert using any fresh fruit in season such as ~

★ Apples

★ Oranges

★ Bananas

★ Pears

★ Kiwi

★ Lilikoi

★ Cherimoya

★ Soursop

★ Dates, chopped

★ Raisins

★ Nuts, chopped

★ Shredded coconut

★ Sprouted trail mix

1) Wash & chop fresh fruit & place in a bowl.

2) Sprinkle with any or all ~ chopped dates, raisins, nuts, shredded coconut & sprouted trail mix.

Dreamboat Dates

This simple dessert blends sweet & salty, yin & yang. It is so quick, easy & satisfying!

★ Medjool dates

★ Macadamia nuts

1) Wash dates & slice lengthwise.

2) Remove pit & replace with a macadamia nut.

Variation ~

★ Replace mac nut with other nuts such as Brazil nuts, hazel nuts, almonds, walnuts & homemade peanut butter. (Recipe is on page 285.)

Aerie's Ginger Joy Balls

★ Dried unsweetened cherries ~ 2 cups

★ Dates pitted ~ 4

★ Pecans ~ 1 cup

★ Fresh ginger ~ 2 or 3 teaspoons

★ Shredded coconut ~ to coat

1) Place dried cherries, pitted dates, pecans & chopped fresh ginger into a food processor.

2) Process until the mixture is a sticky consistency.

3) Roll into balls & coat with shredded coconut.

Raw Cacao Bliss Balls

These bliss balls are outrageously good, so proceed with caution at your own risk!

I find that they give me a burst of energy that enhances productivity & *enthusiasm!*

The word "enthusiasm" comes from the Greek word *"entheos"* which means the God within. It also means to be in ecstasy & Divinely inspired. Enthusiasm is a strength that contributes to physical & mental vitality & well-being. It can be fortified through diet, exercise, mindset, social connection & bliss balls in moderation, among other things.

This recipe makes about 28 bliss balls. They can be stored in the fridge for up to 3 weeks. If they last that long, I admire your self discipline! :)

- ★ Almonds ~ 1 cup
- ★ Walnuts ~ 1 cup
- ★ Medjool dates, **pitted** ~ 2 cups
- ★ Cardamom, freshly ground ~ 1/2 teaspoon (seeds from about15 pods)
- ★ Flax seeds, freshly ground ~ 1 tablespoon
- ★ Raw cacao nibs ~ 3 tablespoons
- ★ Pink Himalayan sea salt ~ a small pinch

1) Remove seeds from cardamom pods & grind in a coffee/seed grinder.

2) Grind flax seeds in a coffee/seed grinder.

3) Place the almonds & walnuts in a food processor first & then add the pitted dates, ground cardamom & ground flax seeds.

4) Process until a sticky consistency ~ pause to scrape down sides, as needed. (It takes a few minutes to release the oils & thoroughly congeal, so I clean up the kitchen while it is processing.)

5) Add the raw cacao nibs & pulse to desired texture.

6) Place the mixture in a bowl & roll into round balls by taking a teaspoonful at a time. Squeeze the mixture in your hand to congeal, then roll gently between both palms to make perfectly round.

Tip ~
1) After grinding the cardamom seeds, stop to breath in the enchanting fragrance!

Variations ~
★ Replace the almonds & walnuts with peanuts & macadamia nuts for a raw cacao peanut butter version. Super yum!
★ Add 1 tablespoon of chia seeds & 1 tablespoon of hemp seeds to amp up your intake of omega-3s & protein! These seeds also add a good texture to the bliss balls.
★ Add freshly ground cloves, cinnamon, nutmeg & fennel for a chai version.
★ Try a batch with just walnuts or a combination of other nuts such as Brazil nuts, pecans, hazel nuts & macadamia nuts.
★ Roll the balls in shredded coconut or finely chopped nuts.

Berry "Blisscream"

Makes a delicious, gorgeous violet color sorbet with no added sugar, preservatives or other junk!

- ★ Frozen pitted cherries ~ 1/2 cup
- ★ Frozen strawberries ~ 1/2 cup
- ★ Frozen blueberries ~ 1/2 cup
- ★ Frozen bananas ~ 6
- ★ Vanilla bean, chopped ~ 1 - 2 inches
- ★ Nuts chopped ~ to garnish
- ★ Raw cacao nibs ~ to garnish
- ★ Fresh mint leaves ~ to garnish

1) Blend in Vitamix or process in juicer until the consistency of sorbet.

2) Garnish with chopped nuts, raw cacao nibs & fresh mint leaves.

Variation ~

- ★ Replace the cherries & blueberries with mango, banana, strawberry & coconut.
- ★ Or make your own creation by combining any frozen fruits that you enjoy together.

Recipes for Delicious & Refreshing Drinks with No Added Sugar, Preservatives or Additives

Ginger Turmeric Tea

This is scientifically shown to be loaded with copious health benefits such as boosting the immune system, reducing inflammation, lowering cholesterol, improving digestion & helping to prevent Alzheimer's disease, just to name a few.

- ★ Fresh ginger ~ 2 - 3 inches
- ★ Fresh turmeric ~ 2 - 3 inches
- ★ Purified water ~ to fill large pot
- ★ Black pepper, optional ~ a dash

1) Boil purified water in a large pot.

2) Wash & scrape or peel fresh ginger root & fresh turmeric root.

3) Slice into thin 'peaces' & add to the pot of water.

4) Add optional dash of black pepper & boil for 20 minutes.

5) Lower heat & simmer until it turns a gorgeous golden-orange color.

Enjoy hot or cold. L'Chaim! (To Life!)

Tip ~

1) Turmeric & black pepper each have health benefits, due to the compounds curcumin & piperine. Some researchers state that with just 1/20 teaspoon or more of black pepper, the bioavailability of turmeric is greatly improved. Some studies indicate that piperine enhances curcumin absorption in the body by up to 2,000%, indicating that combining the spices magnifies their beneficial effects such as reducing inflammation & improving digestion. Other researchers dispute this, so I suggest to experiment & discover what works best for you.

Lemongrass Mint Tea

A refreshing & delicious beverage, pure & simple!

★ Fresh lemongrass ~ 6 stalks
★ Fresh mint leaves ~ 1 cup
★ Purified water

1) Bring a large pot of purified water to boil.

2) Wash fresh lemon grass, add it to the boiling water & boil for about 20 minutes.

3) Wash & detach mint leaves from the stems.

4) Remove pot from heat, add mint leaves & steep.

5) Strain & enjoy hot or cold!

Green Tea with a Squeeze of Fresh Lemon or Lime

Green Tea is loaded with healthy bioactive compounds. Here are just a few of the health benefits ~

- ★ Improves brain function
- ★ Increases fat burning
- ★ Antioxidants lower the risk of some cancers
- ★ Reduces bad breath
- ★ Helps prevent type 2 diabetes
- ★ Helps prevent cardiovascular disease

I use the whole leaves because whole is 'holy'! As I mentioned before, anything commercially ground is inadvertently ground up with insect fragments & other disgusting debris. (Check out the *FDA Food Defect Levels Handbook* to see for yourself, as referenced on page 187.)

Also, the fresh leaves are more potent, fragrant & prana-packed! (*Prana* is a Sanskrit word meaning life-force energy. It is the same as the *Chi* in Tai Chi, the *Ki* in Aikido & the *Mana* in Hawaiian.)

- ★ Whole green tea leaves
- ★ Purified water
- ★ Lemon or lime, freshly squeezed

1) Boil purified water & remove from heat source.

2) Add whole green tea leaves & simmer to desired strength.

3) Add a squeeze of fresh lemon or lime before serving.

4) Enjoy hot or cold.

Variations ~

★ This tea blends well with Ginger Turmeric Tea. (Recipe is on page 305.)

★ Omit the lemon or lime & pour cooled green tea into a jar with a lid. Add a cinnamon stick & place in the fridge overnight. In the morning you will have a delightful cinnamon infused chilled green tea!

Tips ~

1) I like Vahdam Himalayan Signature Green Tea because it is 100% pure green tea. It is mellow, rich & ethically sourced at the foothills of the mighty Himalayas. This company gives back a percentage of their profits to support the wellbeing of their employees. This tea has a delectable flavor of sweet green & vegetal notes in every sip. Smooth, healthy & delicious!

2) Add the used tea leaves to the water that you use to water your plants. It nourishes them!

Homemade Chai Tea

Chai tea is a delicious, fragrant, spicy, invigorating tea loaded with health benefits! It may help boost heart health, reduce blood sugar levels, aid digestion & help with weight loss. Enjoy hot or cold!

★ Fresh ginger & turmeric ~ 2 inch "peace" of each cut into thin slices

★ Cardamom pods ~ 6

★ Cloves, whole ~ 6

★ Fennel &/or anise seeds ~ generous pinch

★ Cinnamon sticks ~ 2

★ Nutmeg ~ 1

★ Star Anise ~ 1

★ Coriander seeds ~ generous pinch

★ Black pepper corns ~ small pinch

★ Green tea leaves ~ 2 teaspoons

1) Fill pot with purified water & bring to a boil.

2) Using a mallet or back of a large spoon, lightly crush the spices.

3) Add all the ingredients except the green tea leaves to the boiling water.

4) Let them boil & then simmer for about 20-30 minutes.

5) Remove from heat & add the green tea leaves.

6) Let simmer until desired potency.

Variations ~

★ Add homemade nut milk. (Recipe is on page 312.)

★ Blend nut milk with dates & vanilla bean. Add to the chai tea for a dessert in a teacup!

Fruit Infusions

A gorgeous violet colored, refreshing, festive, sweet drink with no added sugar, preservatives or other additives! Also, it is great for celebrations in place of wine.

* Strawberries & blueberries ~ (frozen is fine, if you don't have fresh)
* Fresh mint leaves

1) Place washed strawberries, blueberries & fresh mint leaves in a mason jar filled with purified water.

2) Place in fridge overnight & voila, in the morning you have a gorgeous violet fruit infused delicious drink!

Variations ~

* Experiment with other combinations such as dragon fruit (fresh or frozen) with lime, or cucumber & orange, or whatever fresh or frozen organic fruits you have on hand.
* Combine the fruit infusion with Rejuvelac for a non-alcoholic pink 'champagne'!

Rejuvenating Rejuvelac

Rejuvelac is super high in digestive enzymes. It restores a proper balance of probiotics in the gut, helps to improve digestion, boosts immune system & is rich in antioxidants!

* Rye berries ~ 1/2 cup
* Purified water ~ 1/2 gallon jar

1) Soak rye berries in a sprout jar with water overnight or for 8 hours.

2) Drain & rinse sprouts twice a day for a couple days until you see little white tails sprouting.

3) Then fill the jar with purified water & put it in a pantry or cabinet for a couple days until it ferments.

4) Pour off the liquid to drink or refrigerate.

5) The leftover rye berries may be used one or two more times by refilling the jar with purified water.

6) Culture will take about one day after which the seeds may be given to the birds!

Variation ~

★ To give it a yummy flavor, mix the Rejuvelac, half & half, with the ginger turmeric tea or a fruit infusion when you are ready to drink it.
(Recipe for ginger turmeric tea is on page 305 & the recipe for infusions is on page 310.)

Homemade Almond Milk

Homemade almond milk is free of preservatives & is high in protein, fiber & potassium. It is a great replacement for dairy milk as well as store bought plant milks.

It can be used for cooking, baking, pouring over cereal, smoothies, etc.

Soaking almonds makes them softer, less bitter, easier to digest & makes it easier to absorb some nutrients. It is preferable to soak them over night or for 8 hours, however less time is still beneficial.

Almond milk can be made in a juicer, Vitamix or high-powered blender.

In a juicer ~

★ Almonds ~ 2 cups
★ Purified water ~ 2 cups

1) Soak almonds in water for 8 hours.

2) Rinse the almonds.

3) Alternate feeding the almonds & equal parts of water into the juicer.

4) Enjoy!

In a Vitamix ~

★ Almonds ~ 1 cup
★ Purified water ~ 3 cups
★ Dates, pitted ~ 2 (optional)

1) Soak almonds in water for 8 hours.

2) Rinse the almonds.

3) Blend almonds & water.

4) For a more refined smooth texture, strain in a nut bag or a fine mesh sieve.

Variations ~

★ Blend with cinnamon, nutmeg, cardamom, vanilla bean & a pinch of salt.
★ Replace almonds with other nuts such as cashews, pecans, macadamia nuts or a combination thereof.

Golden Turmeric Almond Milk

The spices in this nurturing golden, glowing 'meal in a teacup' are loaded with copious health benefits & may help to ~

- ★ Reduce inflammation & joint pain
- ★ Improve memory & brain function
- ★ Protect against heart disease
- ★ Reduce risk of cancer
- ★ Lower blood sugar levels
- ★ The curcumin in turmeric may help to improve mood
- ★ These ingredients contain antibacterial, antiviral & antifungal properties

- ★ Almond milk ~ 1cup (recipe is on page 312)
- ★ Turmeric, minced ~ 1/4 teaspoon
- ★ Ginger, minced ~ 1/4 teaspoon
- ★ Medjool dates, pitted ~ 3
- ★ Clove ~ small fragment of one whole clove (use sparingly or it will dominate the flavor)
- ★ Fennel seeds, whole ~ small pinch
- ★ Cinnamon, freshly ground ~ small pinch (see page 224)
- ★ Nutmeg, freshly ground ~ small pinch (see page 224)
- ★ Cardamom seeds ~ small pinch
- ★ Black pepper ~ small pinch

1) Wash, peel & mince small "peace" of ginger & turmeric.

2) Remove cardamom seeds from the pod.

3) Place almond milk in a Vitamix or high-powered blender.

4) Add all the ingredients & blend until a warm golden color.

5) Enjoy warmed up, room temperature or cold.

Variation ~

★ For a burst of energy, add some raw cacao nibs & blend thoroughly!

Goddess Lemon - 'aid'

This is my unprocessed version of the *Master Cleanse* which is typically made with lemon juice, maple syrup & cayenne. I have named my *unprocessed* version the *Goddess Cleanse*.

This can be used as a cleanse to give your organs a rest from digesting solid foods or as a refreshing, delicious beverage!

Lemon-aid, 'aids' your health in many ways such as ~

★ Promotes hydration

★ Good source of vitamin C

★ Supports weight loss

★ Improves your skin quality

★ Aids digestion

★ Freshens breath

★ Helps prevent kidney stones

★ Alkalizes the system

Lemon juice in its natural state is acidic with a pH of about 2, but once metabolized it actually becomes alkaline with a pH well above 7. So, outside the body, anyone can see that lemon juice is very acidic. However, once fully digested, its effect is proven to be alkalizing with many health benefits.

As I mentioned earlier, lemon juice can affect the enamel on your teeth, so I recommend drinking it with a reusable straw to bypass the teeth. It is also a good practice to rinse your mouth with purified water after drinking lemon-aid to remove any residual acidity.

* Fresh lemon ~ 1
* Dates, pitted ~ 3 - 5
* Red chili pepper ~ 1 (deseeded, unless you like it super hot!)
* Purified water ~ to fill the blender

1) Cut a fresh lemon into quarters. Remove the peel & seeds.

2) Place the lemon in a Vitamix or high-powered blender with the pitted dates, deseeded red chili pepper & purified water.

3) Blend & enjoy!

Variations ~
* After blending, add a few mint leaves.
* Add a slice of fresh ginger &/or fresh turmeric.
* Add a cinnamon stick to the jar.

Angel's Cinnamon Water

So simple & so delicious without any added sugar or other junk!

Cinnamon has been prized for its medicinal properties for thousands of years & modern science has now confirmed what people have known for ages. Cinnamon is loaded with antioxidants. It has anti-inflammatory properties, helps to fight bacterial & fungal infections, may reduce the risk of heart disease & cancer, can lower blood sugar levels & has a plethora of other impressive health benefits!

★ Cinnamon stick ~ 1
★ Purified water ~ 1 quart jar

1) Rinse cinnamon stick & place in quart jar filled with purified water.

2) Place covered jar in fridge overnight & voila, in the morning you have this flavorful ambrosia!

Variations ~

★ Pour cooled green tea into a jar with a lid. Add a cinnamon stick to the jar & place in the fridge overnight. In the morning you will have a delightful, cinnamon infused chilled green tea!
★ Replace cinnamon with cardamom & make refreshing, delicious, cardamon water or combine both!

Tip ~

1) You can refill the jar with purified water several times with the same cinnamon stick! This is a beverage you will want to "stick" with! :)

Happy Independence Day, Every Day!

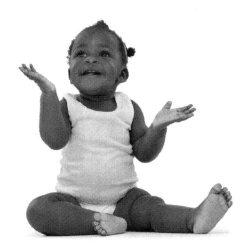

"For to be free is not merely to cast off one's chains, but to live in a way that respects & enhances the freedom of others."
- Nelson Mandela

Today is the 4th of July & I am celebrating Independence Day by working on this book. In so doing, I came across this *Declaration for Independence for Animals* by PETA (People for Ethical Treatment of Animals) that I would like to share with you.

Regardless of when you read this book, these inalienable rights hold true for all living beings. Animal liberation leads to environmental liberation, which leads to human, political & economic liberation, which leads to spiritual liberation.

Declaration of Independence for Animals from *PETA*

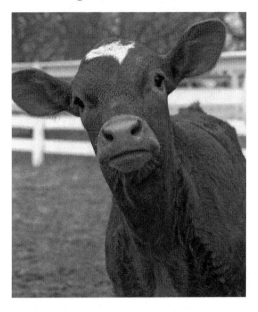

"All individuals are entitled to certain liberties as their birthright, whether they were born an orca, a macaque, a chicken or a bat.

We hold these truths to be self-evident, that no human being is entitled to use perceived difference as justification for robbing a sentient individual of his or her inalienable right to freedom, dignity, autonomy, the pursuit of happiness and the avoidance of needless pain and suffering.

Therefore, we have conceived this declaration of the rights of all animals.

Animals have the right not to be used in experiments, as food, as clothing, as entertainment, or in any other way against their own best interests.

Animals, including mice, who can solve complex puzzles with remarkable speed, have the right not to be imprisoned in laboratory cages and burned, poisoned, shocked, or mutilated.

Animals, including barn owls, who have been known to share their nests with animals of other species, have the right not to be used in any experiment.

Animals, including pigs, who have frequently saved the lives of their human guardians, have the right not to be crammed by the thousands into filthy, windowless sheds.

Animals, including fish, many of whom rub against one another as a sign of affection, have the right not to be impaled on a hook or caught in a net and pulled out of the water to suffocate.

Animals, including chickens, who worry about the future and pass knowledge down from one generation to the next, have the right not to have their throats slit and to die in terror in a slaughterhouse.

Animals, including rabbits, who leap in the air when they feel joyful, have the right not to have their skin torn off.

Animals, including sheep, who can read emotions on each other's faces, have the right not to have their protective covering sliced off.

Animals, including orcas, whose pods each has its own language, have the right not to be taken from their homes, forcibly bred and held captive in a concrete pool or behind bars in a cage.

Animals, including elephants, who can empathize with others' pain, have the right not to be beaten, shackled and forced to perform demeaning tricks.

Animals, including geese, who often spend the remainder of their life as a widow or widower after their lifelong mate is killed, have the right not to be shot for "sport."

Animals, including raccoons, who frequently "wash" their food in water, have the right not to be killed just because humans have taken over their habitat and don't want them there.

Animals, including pigeons, who can recognize all 26 letters of the English alphabet, have the right not to be harassed and harmed just for trying to survive.

Animals have the right to live, to raise families, to explore, to make choices and to spend their time pursuing their own interests, not those of humans.

Animals have repeatedly appealed to humans' sensibilities and objected to our tyranny over them by fleeing, hiding, crying out, or fighting for their lives, most often to no avail.

All living beings experience hope, joy, love, fear, pain, loss, and sorrow, and we hold that all individuals are deserving of respect and consideration.

In conclusion, animals have the right to be free of the crushing grip of human oppression, and we must grant them their independence."
- PETA

As Albert Schweitzer said, "*Until he extends his circle of compassion to include all living things, man will not himself find peace.*"

As Meenakshi Angel Honig said, "*When we extend lovingkindness to all, our true nature of peace will remain undisturbed.*"

May the true treasure of peace reign supreme for one & all!

Conclusion ~ The Power of Love

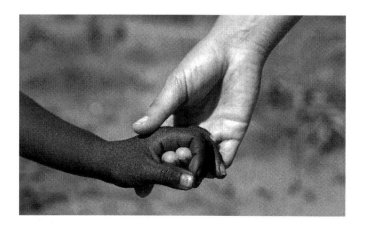

"The pure love of one soul can offset the hatred of millions."
- Mahatma Gandhi

It takes about 242,000 rose petals to distill approximately 5mL of rose oil. 5mL is equal to 0.17 fluid ounces. I have done my best to be a distiller, to address a vast topic & distill it down to the key points & connect the dots that I have shared with you in this book.

As Dr. Martin Luther King, Jr. said, *"Power without love is reckless and abusive, and love without power is sentimental & anemic. Power at its best is love implementing the demands of justice, and justice at its best is power correcting everything that stands against love."*

Love is our true nature. When someone performs an act of kindness, serotonin, a good feeling hormone is released. Serotonin is not only released in the person offering the act of kindness, but also in the person who is receiving the act of kindness, as well as in anyone witnessing the act of kindness.

The goal of all goals is to feel good. When we feel good, we have our best to give & everyone wins. That is why, as it says in the Talmud,

"Kindness is the highest form of wisdom."

(A friend of mine, who was proofreading for me, pointed out that for some people the goal of all goals is to serve God regardless of how they feel. Just to clarify, why would anyone want to serve God? It is because he or she believes that in so doing they will feel good. So ultimately even our 'selfless' actions are an attempt to feel good.)

In the Yoga way of thinking, 108 is an auspicious number. So, in conclusion, I would like to summarize by offering you ~

108 Benefits of Going Vegan!

1) Relieve animal suffering

2) Eliminate starvation worldwide

3) Reverse water shortage

4) Reverse deforestation

5) Reduce Amazon fires (forests are burned & cleared for GMO soy for livestock)

6) Prevent desertification

7) Reduce pollution

8) Save our seas

9) Reduce reliance on fossil fuels

10) Reduce global warming

11) Reverse the climate crisis

12) Reduce your carbon footprint

13) Prevent dead zones in the ocean

14) Increase energy

15) Live more in harmony with nature

16) Improve your health
17) Lower risk of heart disease by 40%
18) Reverse heart disease (check out *Reversing Heart Disease* by Dr. Dean Ornish)
19) Lower risk of cancer
20) Reverse type 2 diabetes
21) Decrease allergies
22) Get more fiber
23) Improve digestion, assimilation & elimination
24) Shed excess weight
25) Have better gut health
26) Lower blood sugar level
27) Improve kidney function
28) Reduce pain from arthritis
29) Have more balanced hormones
30) Lower your cholesterol
31) Get rid of acne (linked to dairy products)
32) Have more vitality
33) Increase sexual virility
34) Improve athletic performance
35) Get better sleep by saving sheep instead of counting them
36) Live in congruence with your values of kindness
37) Reduce cognitive dissonance
38) Free yourself from antidepressants
39) Improve your mood

40) Enjoy more peace of mind
41) Experience more inner calm
42) Eliminate PTSD for over 500,000 slaughterhouse workers
43) Discover new foods & amazing recipes
44) Be a positive role model
45) Experience a kinship with all animals
46) Help shed light on human supremacy & speciesism
47) Eliminate cruel animal testing
48) Contribute to reversing antibiotic resistance caused by animal agriculture
49) Prevent future pandemics & other zoonotic infectious diseases
50) Contribute to the evolution of human consciousness
51) Be an instrument of lovingkindness
52) Prevent extinction of species
53) Be a compassionate presence on Earth
54) Improve mental clarity
55) Happier conscience
56) Healthier relationships
57) Reduce modern day slavery
58) Reverse environmental racism
59) Heighten awareness for others
60) Be a more sustainable consumer
61) Support conscious businesses that are based on kindness & sustainability

62) Eliminate using crushed beetles for pigment in conventional lipstick
63) Support vegan businesses such as *100% Pure* lipstick that use pigment from fruit instead of crushed insects
64) Enjoy healthier plant-based skin care products
65) Have glowing skin & a glowing heart
66) Be more youthful (a vegan diet is rich in antioxidants & phytonutrients)
67) Enjoy & support healthier non-toxic vegan household products
68) Eliminate the cruel & polluting leather industry
69) Support vegan leather made from food waste such as *No Saints* & *Louis Vuitton* vegan leather sneakers
70) Promote vegan fashion items made from plastic waste by companies such as *Thies* & *Insecta*
71) Reduce plastic waste by purchasing vegan shoes such as *Adidas* who teamed up with *Parley for the Oceans* to produce vegan shoes with plastic pulled from the ocean
72) Help save our oceans by choosing vegan products because each shoe contains 12 plastic bottles worth of waste, with some of this coming from discarded fishing nets
73) Support sustainable industries such as leather made out of pineapple leaf fibers, apple peals & plastic trash pulled from the ocean
74) Eliminate the unbelievably cruel wool industry
75) Support vegan alternatives such as hemp, linen, organic cotton, bamboo, seaweed & wood to make cruelty-free clothing
76) Eliminate the cruel silk industry by choosing vegan silk

77) Let birds keep their feathers & don't go down with the cruel down industry, by choosing the many wonderful vegan alternatives

78) Contribute to social justice in all areas

79) Be an agent of positive change

80) Open up to higher levels of consciousness

81) Enjoy deeper meditations

82) Enjoy a more flexible body temple because it is not filled with toxins

83) Be a living example of *ahimsa* (non-violence)

84) Set a precedent for reforming other forms of domination & violence

85) Contribute to eradicating "herd mentality"

86) Sharpen your critical thinking skills & discernment capabilities

87) Save the bees

88) Support ethical honey made out of apples & sweet potatoes

89) Enjoy clean renewed taste buds

90) Fresher breath

91) Smell better

92) Boost immunity

93) Increase disease-fighting antioxidants

94) Have stronger bones (100 grams of kale contains more calcium than 100 grams of milk)

95) Decrease risk of death by 20% (2018 study in *The Lancet*)

96) Be more productive (*American Journal of Health*)

97) Have better concentration

98) Improve sensory acuity

99) Save thousands of animals over the years

100) Save your mind, body, heart & Soul

101) Help shift consciousness from cruelty to lovingkindness

102) Live longer

103) Save Planet Earth

104) Pave the way of Lovingkindness for future generations!

105) Be on the right side of history

106) It's the right thing to do!

107) Good Karma ~ What goes around comes around

108) Add your own! :)

Given that 72 billion animals & over a trillion sea creatures are tortured & killed every year & given all of the detrimental ramifications of that, which I have outlined in my *10 compelling reasons to choose a plant-based diet*, it is crystal clear that going vegan is the conscionable choice & *the Soulution* to all of the major problems that we face on planet Earth today.

I hope & pray that you take this to heart, implement it in your life & share it with one & all. We can't do everything but we can each do something.

John Lewis, the dedicated civil rights leader & US congressman, was known as the conscience of the congress. He ascended from his physical body while I was writing this book, on July 17, 2020 at the age of 80.

He wrote this essay shortly before his death & it is so applicable to what I have shared with you in this book.

"Though I may not be here with you, I urge you to answer the highest calling of your heart and stand up for what you truly believe. In my life I have done all I can to demonstrate that the way of peace, the way of love and nonviolence is the more excellent way. Now it is your turn to let freedom ring. When historians pick up their pens to write the story of the 21st century, let them say that it was your generation who laid down the heavy burdens of hate at last and that peace finally triumphed over violence, aggression and war. So, I say to you, walk with the wind, brothers and sisters, and let the spirit of peace and the power of everlasting love be your guide."
- John Lewis

When *the spirit of peace & the power of everlasting love* guides our dietary choices, it has a positive impact on every aspect of life on Earth & beyond!

As Joseph Campbell said, *"The privilege of a lifetime is being who you are."*

So, would you rather be an agent of horrific cruelty or be on the right side of history & go vegan?

"To delay justice is injustice." - William Penn

"Do not be daunted by the enormity of the world's grief. Do justly, now. Love mercy, now. Walk humbly, now. You are not obligated to complete the work, but neither are you free to abandon it."
- The Talmud

"Do what you can, with what you have, where you are."
- Theodore Roosevelt

I invite & encourage you with all of my heart to be part of **The Soulution**. Together we can make Planet Earth a Vegan Heavenly Body!

*You don't need any other reason,
or any other season, to Go Vegan!*

Here is my version of Michael Jackson's song ~

ABC, it's easy as 123
As simple as Do, Re, Mi
ABC, 123
Go Vegan Baby, You & Me!

& as the Beatles sang,

"And in the end, the love you take is equal to the love you make!"

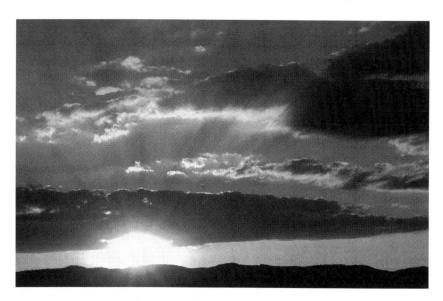

Soli Deo Gloria ~ All Glory to God

Even self - effort is Grace

Resources to Have & to Share!

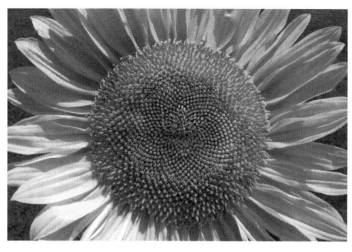

"The secret of change is to focus all of your energy, not on fighting the old, but on building the new."
- Socrates

There are tons of resources readily available to support you in your plant-based diet & lifestyle. Here are a few documentaries, books, websites, YouTube channels, phone apps & Meet-up groups that I highly recommend to get started.

You can also use these resources to inform & inspire your family, friends, community & world. For example, how about having a movie night with air popped popcorn with your family & friends. Then discuss afterwards what touched each person the most & one specific step they are committed to taking to move toward a plant-based diet & lifestyle. If they are already a vegan, ask them one specific step they will take to spread the word.

Or form a book club utilizing the books below such as, *The World Peace Diet, Vegan in 30 Days,* or this book to discuss, inspire & encourage each other to choose a healthy plant-based diet & share the same with one & all!

Having a vegan potluck is a great way to share the message in a fun, loving, nurturing, yummy & creative way!

The best way to learn is to teach. Consider being a vegan mentor for others who are just getting started. It is great to share your experience, favorite recipes, resources & support with others.

What goes around, comes around. I have noticed that when I support others, support comes to me in whatever area I need it & when I need it.

I remember saying to a dear friend, *"I have learned that service positions us for Grace."* She responded by saying, *"Service **is** Grace!"*

I refer to this as, *"The Magic of the unseen hand."* Tap into it & see for yourself!

Documentaries

- ★ Forks over Knives
- ★ Earthlings
- ★ Dominion
- ★ Cowspiracy
- ★ What the Health
- ★ The Game Changers
- ★ Vegucated

- ★ Food, Inc.
- ★ Fat, Sick & Nearly Dead
- ★ Live & Let Live
- ★ Food Matters
- ★ Blackfish
- ★ Babe
- ★ Meat the Truth
- ★ Simply Raw: Reversing Diabetes in 30 Days
- ★ Hungry for Change
- ★ Plant Pure Nation
- ★ H.O.P.E.: What You Eat Matters
- ★ The End of Meat
- ★ Seaspiracy

Books

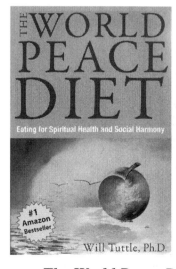
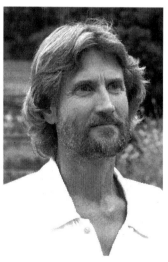

The World Peace Diet by Dr. Will Tuttle

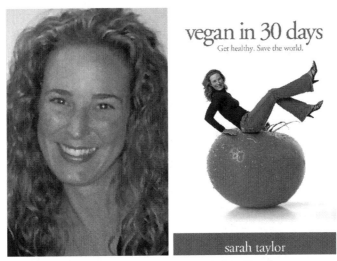

Vegan in 30 Days by Sarah Taylor

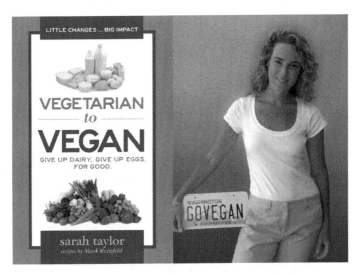

Vegetarian to Vegan by Sarah Taylor

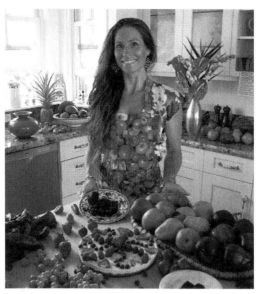

*Incredibly Delicious - Recipes for A New Paradigm
& Body Temple Gourmet* by Brook Le'amohala

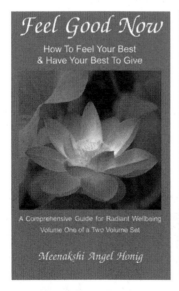
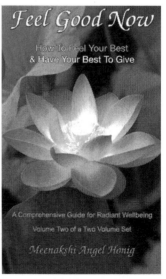

*Feel Good Now ~ How to Feel Your Best
& Have Your Best to Give*
Volume One & Volume Two
by Meenakshi Angel Honig

Books Continued

- *Diet for a New America* by John Robbins
- *How Not to Die* by Dr. Michael Greger
- *Reversing Heart Disease* by Dr. Dean Ornish
- *The China Study* by Dr. T. Colin Campbell
- *Why We Love Dogs, Eat Pigs, & Wear Cows* by Dr. Melanie Joy
- *Healthy at 100* by John Robbins
- *Breaking the Food Seduction* by Dr. Neal Barnard
- *Eat to Live* by Dr. Joel Fuhrman
- *Green for Life* by Victoria Boutenko
- *Vegan: The Ethics of Eating* by Erik Marcus
- *The Pleasure Trap* by Dr. Doug Lisle & Dr. Alan Goldhamer
- *Slaughterhouse* by Gail Eisnitz
- *That's Why We Don't Eat Animals* by Ruby Roth

Websites

- Dr. Will Tuttle - www.worldpeacediet.com
- Dr. Dean Ornish - www.ornish.com
- Dr. Michael Klaper - www.doctorklaper.com
- Dr. Michael Greger - www.nutritionfacts.org
- Dr. Joel Fuhrman - www.drfuhrman.com
- Dr. Neal Barnard - www.pcrm.org
- Dr. Michael McDougall - www.drmcdougall.com
- Dr. Sandra McLanahan - www.yogaville.org

- ★ PETA - www.peta.org
- ★ Fully Raw Kristina - www.fullyraw.com
- ★ Sarah Taylor - www.facebook.com/The-Vegan-Next-Door-115947898461766/
- ★ Fredrick Swaroop Honig - www.thegardens.org
- ★ Rebecca McLean - www.colci.org
- ★ Meenakshi Angel Honig - www.angelyoga.com

Vegan Phone Apps

★ **Is it Vegan?** - www.isitvegan.net ~ Analyzes ingredients & lets you know if the product is vegan. Food manufacturers make it complicated; this app makes it simple.

★ **Happy Cow** - www.happycow.net ~ Awesome way to find vegan food in 183 countries.

★ **Forks Over Knives** - apps.apple.com/us/app/forks-over-knives-healthy/id903911740 ~ Great Recipes

★ **Vanilla Bean** - play.google.com/store/apps/details?id=de.grunzeug.vanillabeanandhl=en ~ Tasty Vegan Restaurants

★ **Food Monster** - www.onegreenplanet.org/foodmonster/ ~ Vegan & allergy friendly recipes

★ **Dr. Greger's Daily Dozen** - play.google.com/store/apps/details?id=org.nutritionfacts.dailydozenandhl=en ~ List of healthiest foods

★ **Yelp** - play.google.com/store/apps/details?id=com.yelp.androidandhl=en ~ Vegan friendly restaurants in your area

★ **Air Vegan** - apps.apple.com/us/app/airvegan/id1265851834 ~ Airport eateries with vegan options

★ **Gonutss** - www.gonutss.com ~ Vegan Translator provides amazing alternatives for eggs, desserts, milk, protein, iron, meat, etc.

* **Vegan Explanatory Card** - www.maxlearning.net/HEALth/V-Cards.pdf ~ These V-Cards explain the needs of a vegan diet in 83 different languages!

* **VegWeb** - www.vegweb.com ~ 13,000 5-star recipes

* **Cruelty Free** - apps.apple.com/us/app/cruelty-free/id313825734 ~ From household products to a new lipstick, consult this app to make sure you are only buying cruelty-free items.

* **Meet Up** - www.meetup.com ~ Great way to meet vegans or start your own vegan meet-up group.

Yummy Vegan Recipes
* www.vegweb.com - Making vegan easy
* www.fatfreevegan.com - Fat-free vegan recipes
* www.drfuhrman.com - Vegan recipes galore
* http://www.bodytemplegourmet.com - Vegan culinary conscious bliss
* www.drmcdougall.com - Bountiful vegan recipe archives
* www.pcrm.org - Vegan recipes including weight-loss recipes
* www.worldpeacediet.com/cooking-videos/ - Madeleine's Intuitive Kitchen Sumptuous vegan recipes & YouTube demonstrations
* www.fullyraw.com - Colorful, outrageously delicious raw vegan recipes
* www.sproutman.com - Great recipes incorporating fresh sprouts
* www.Zalad.live - Ziggy's Zalad

About Meenakshi Angel Honig

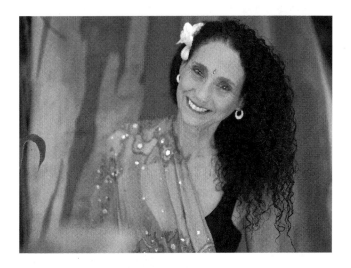

Meenakshi Angel Honig is dedicated to peace & lovingkindness. She has studied with the world-renowned, highly revered & deeply loved Yoga Master, His Holiness, Sri Swami Satchidananda since the age of 16.

Meenakshi Angel is an internationally acclaimed certified Integral Yoga Instructor & Yoga Teacher Trainer with nearly 50 years of teaching experience, including television instruction.

She served as the premier Mind, Body, Spirit, Yoga Instructor & Stress Management Consultant at the award-winning Grand Wailea Resort for over 17 years & she currently teaches at the spectacular five-star Fairmont Kea Lani on Maui.

Meenakshi Angel is a licensed minister & an animal rights advocate. She is a highly respected leader in promoting plant-based nutrition for individual & global wellbeing.

Meenakshi Angel has produced 5 DVDs, 2 CDs & is the author of 11 books.

Her work is endorsed by Sri Swami Satchidananda, Dr. Wayne Dyer, Dr. Deepak Chopra, Dr. Dean Ornish, Dr. Joel Fuhrman, Dr. Michael Klaper, Dr. John Gray, Dr. Will Tuttle, John Robins, Alan Cohen, Marci Schimoff, Katherine Woodward Thomas, Miranda Macpherson, Swami Karunananda, Mirabai Devi & many other great luminaries!

To find out more about how you can benefit from Meenakshi Angel's services & products, please visit ~

www.AngelYoga.com

Connect with Angel in Hawaii, in Your Area, or Online

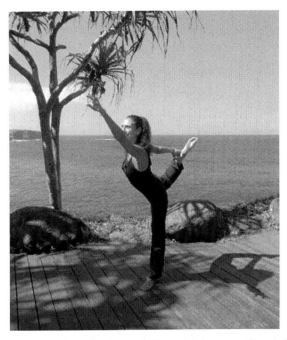

Meenakshi Angel Honig currently resides on the splendorous Hawaiian Island of Maui, where she conducts Programs, Classes, Private Sessions, Personalized Retreats & Yoga Teacher Certification Courses.

Programs, Speaking Engagements & Book Signings can be arranged in your area, as well.

Meenakshi Angel is also a licensed Minister in the state of Hawaii & would be happy to perform your Wedding & Personalized Ceremonies.

Sessions are available by appointment, in person, on the phone & on Skype.

Meenakshi Angel is happy to tailor a Program to meet & exceed your needs & dreams!

**To Arrange Group & Private Instruction
on Maui, in Your Area, or Online in ~**

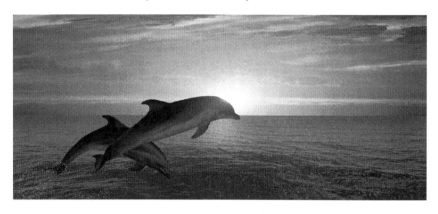

- ★ Yoga & Meditation
- ★ Mastering Stress & Lifestyle Design
- ★ Goals Clarification & Implementation
- ★ Plant-based Nutrition Tailored for You
- ★ Healthy Back & Strong Core
- ★ Transformational Life Coaching
- ★ Clear Your Life ~ Clearing Clutter on All Levels
- ★ Guided Glorious Nature Adventures
- ★ Personalized Rejuvenation Retreats
- ★ Yoga Teachers Certification Courses
- ★ Writing Retreats
- ★ Cleansing & Juicing Retreats
- ★ Licensed Weddings
- ★ Personalized Ceremonies in Paradise

Please Contact ~ Meenakshi Angel Honig
www.AngelYoga.com
Angel@AngelYoga.com
808 - 573 - 1414 (Voicemail only)

Products to Serve your Wellbeing
by Meenakshi Angel Honig

DVDs or MP4 Digital Files

★ Yoga Feels Good ~ 1-Hour $25

★ Yoga Feels Good ~ 30 Minute Yoga Tune-up $25

★ Seven Techniques for Mastering Stress $25

★ Seven Easy Steps for a Healthy Back & Strong Core .. $25

★ Ten Compelling Reasons to Choose a Plant-based Diet ... $25

CDs or MP3 Digital File

★ Relaxation & Affirmations for Radiant Wellbeing $20

Books

★ Drops of Nectar ~ Loving Reminders $10

★ 108 Ways to Feel Better $10

★ 108 Jokes to Bring a Smile to Your Heart $10

★ 108 Jewels of Wisdom $10

★ 108 Ways to Free Yourself from Pain $10

★ 108 Ways to Say I Love $10

★ Sweet Remembrance $10

★ Feel Good Now ~ Black & White $25
   Color Volume One $49
   Color Volume Two $49
   Color E-book per Volume $10

★ The Soulution: 10 Compelling Reasons to Choose
a Plant-based Diet & Lifestyle - The Why & The How

Black & White... $25
Color... $49
Color E-book... $10

Please use PayPal on Meenakshi Angel's website ~
www.AngelYoga.com

Or make checks payable to ~

Wellbeing International

P. O. Box 2300

Kihei, Maui, HI 96753

Telephone (808) 573-1414 (Voicemail only)

Thank you for your order & Enjoy!

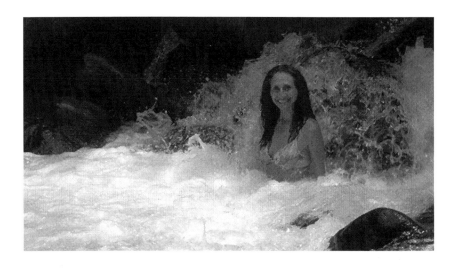

Sending You a Waterfall of Happy Blessings! ~ Angel

This Book is Dedicated with Love & Gratitude To ~

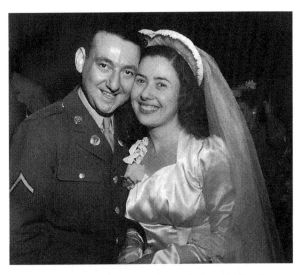

My Beloved Parents, Jean & Jacob Honig

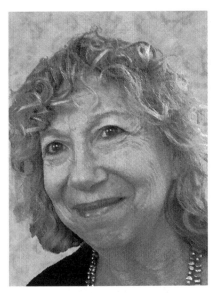

My Beloved Sister,
Jiya Kowarsky

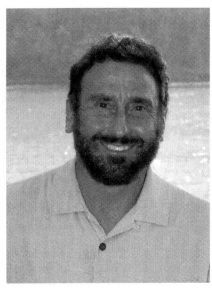

My Beloved Brother,
Swaroop Fredrick Honig

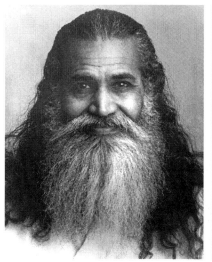

My Beloved Gurudev,
Sri Swami Satchidananda

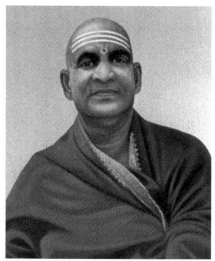

My Beloved Grand Guru,
Master Sivananda

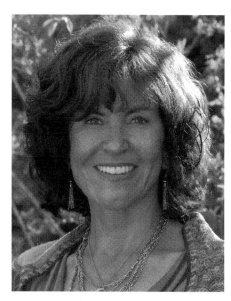

My Beloved BFF
& Purpose Partner, Rebecca McLean

I would not be who I am, or have the ability to give what I give, without their love, support & encouragement. It is upon their shoulders, I stand.

"I am everything I am because you loved me!"

May the merit that is generated from this book,
bring infinite blessings to their noble Souls, here, now & eternally!

Photo by Julie Stuehser

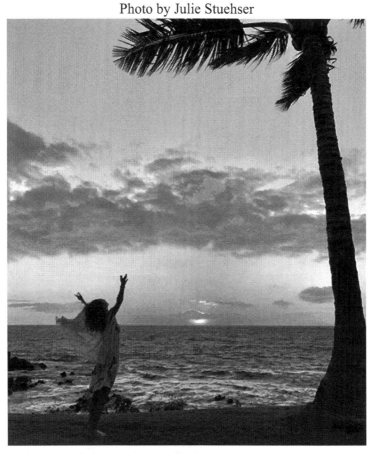

Meenakshi Angel Honig, Maui Hawaii

**May All be Blessed with Peace, Comfort,
Lovingkindness, Bliss & Enlightenment!**

Made in the USA
Columbia, SC
22 July 2023